PRAISE FOR BAD RHYMES, NO REASON

Simon's newest work, *Bad Rhymes, No Reason*, provides a genuine glimpse into the experience of stroke recovery that is valuable for patients and loved ones alike. Simon's light-hearted and earnest perspective reflects an optimistic realism that is so important for resilience in the face of life's adversity. And the book's illustrations are so charming!

Melissa D. Stockbridge, Ph.D., CCC-SLP
Johns Hopkins University, Baltimore, MD

Bad Rhymes, No Reason gives us a glimpse into the many challenges faced by someone surviving a right brain stroke. Through his open and honest essays and his delightful poems, Barton gives us a poignant glimpse into his new life post-stroke. He shares stories of therapists, nurses, and other stroke survivors he has met along the way, and introduces us to Sarah, his devoted care partner. He illustrates the long and winding road to recovery and leaves us feeling hopeful that new friendships, improved function, and acceptance are the rewards for the hard work and perseverance that stroke recovery requires!

Melissa Johnson, Ph.D., CCC-SLP
Nazareth College, Rochester, NY

Simon Barton's newest book, *Bad Rhymes, No Reason*, is a heartfelt, witty, well-written exploration of the many different facets to stroke recovery, like relationships, self-image, work/career, and love and loss. As a stroke and aphasia researcher, I found myself growing in my understanding of how these factors interact with recovery, guided by beautiful prose and equally charming illustrations. This is a delightful read that keeps you guessing as to what's coming next and also makes you appreciate the bravery and creativity of its writer.

Brielle C Stark, PhD
Indiana University, Bloomington, IN

Simon Barton's reflections on his experience of life after a right hemisphere stroke is an honest and at times moving personal narrative. *Bad Rhymes, No Reason* takes the reader on a journey that offers insights into the factors that influence the very individual response to loss caused by a significant health event. FAIR is indeed a powerful word as are the people encountered on our path that help us to shift our perspectives. A book with something for both those affected by stroke and health professionals alike.

Ronelle Hewetson, PhD
Griffiths University, Gold Coast, Queensland, Australia

When you hear the word "stroke" many people think, "that's it...life is over." Simon Barton's book of poems and essays, *Bad Rhymes, No Reason*, is uplifting and witty. It demonstrates that life for someone with a stroke isn't over; it is just different. I especially loved Simon's ability to share his ups and downs through his writing. It is inspiring, and I look forward to reading more from him!

Holly Hanley, Ph.D., CCC-SLP
Appalachian State University, Boone, NC

Bad Rhymes, No Reason

By Simon C. Barton
Illustrated by Sarah C. Hardy

Also published by Simon Barton

Not so Green as Cabbage Looking: Recovering from a Stroke with a Little Gallows Humor Along the Way

BAD RHYMES, NO REASON

Reflections, Ramblings & Rantings of a Rancorous Stroke Survivor

By Simon C. Barton
Illustrated by Sarah C. Hardy

MOUNTAIN PAGE PRESS
Hendersonville, NC

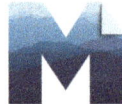

Published 2022 by Mountain Page Press

Hardcover ISBN 978-1-952714-55-9
Paperback ISBN 978-1-952714-56-6

Copyright © 2022 Simon C. Barton
All rights reserved.
No part of this publication may be reproduced, stored in a retrieval system, distributed or transmitted in any form or by any means (electronic, mechanical, photocopying, recording, or otherwise) without prior written permission from the publisher.

For information, contact the publisher at:
Mountain Page Press
Hendersonville, NC

Visit: www.mountainpagepress.com

Written by Simon C. Barton
Illustrated by Sarah C. Hardy

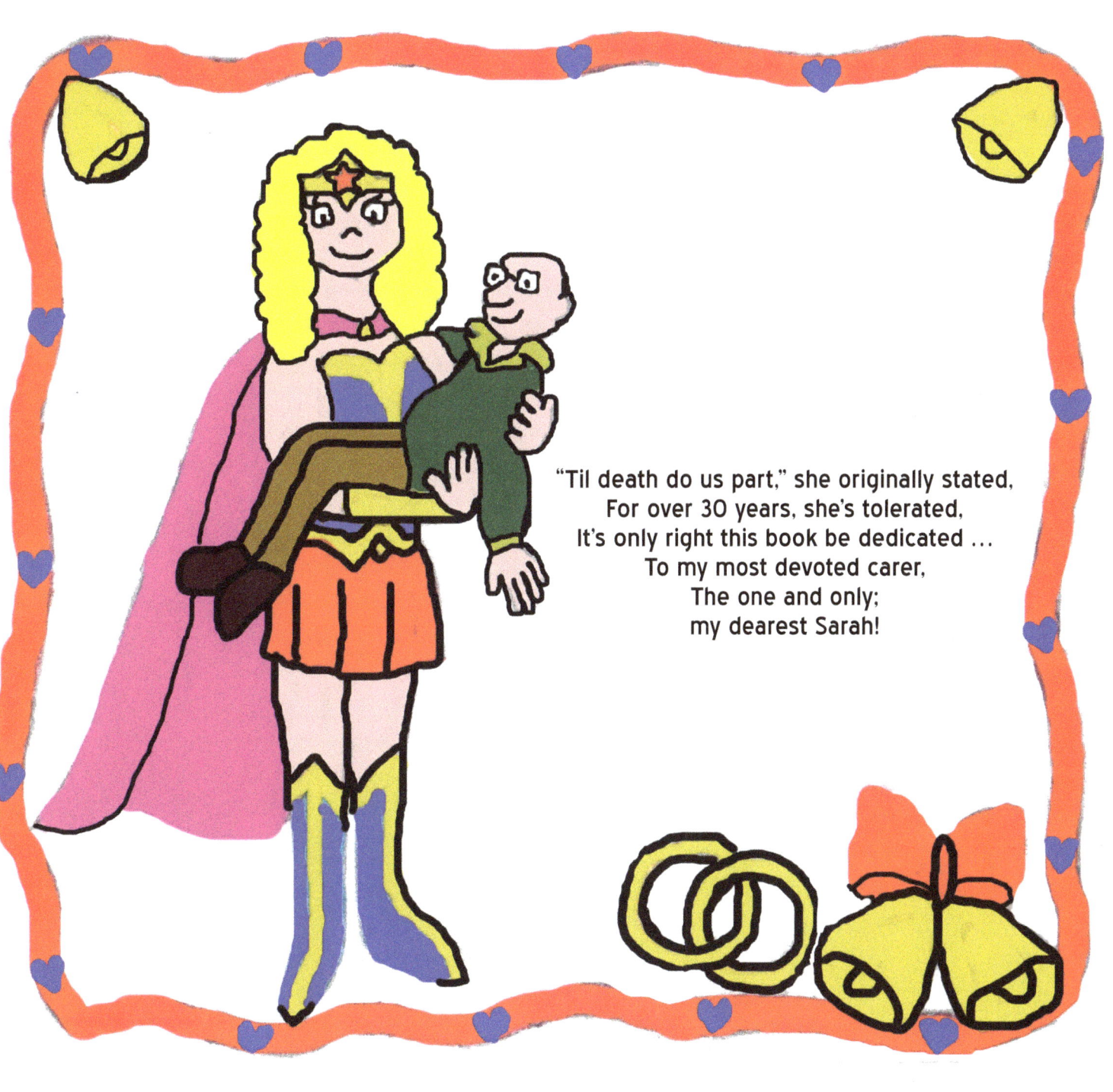

"Til death do us part," she originally stated,
For over 30 years, she's tolerated,
It's only right this book be dedicated ...
To my most devoted carer,
The one and only;
my dearest Sarah!

TABLE OF CONTENTS

1. Aspiring Poet 6
2. Simon's Story 9
3. The Journey 11
4. Angels 13
5. The Therapist 16
6. Aphasia 19
7. Heaven and Hell 22
8. Term of Endearment 25
9. What's Your Name Again? 28
10. Ahead of My Time 31
11. Reticence 33
12. My Mate Keith 35
13. Just a Glimpse 38
14. Rotten Endings 42
15. Murder Mystery Mayhem 44
16. Life's Quarterly Highlights 47
17. Neuro Fatigue 49
18. Inspiration 51
19. Oh to Sing 53
20. The Cantata 56
21. Another 4-Letter F-Word 58
22. Fog 62
23. Mr. Darcy 64
24. Hellhound 68
25. Reverent Reflection 70
26. When It Rains 72
27. Grampsi's Law 74
28. Cavalry of The Clouds 76
29. Young at Heart 80
30. Fairest of Ladies 82
31 Better than the Rest 85
32. Trouble and Strife 87
33. Something 89
34. Wind in my Sails 92
35. Neuroplasticity 95
36. Very Best of Men 97
37. Etiquette 99
38. You Know You're Old 102
39. Mousse Attack 105
40. Big Mr. Muffet 107
41. Break A Leg 109
42. Sixteen 113
43. No News Today 117
44. Ethel and the Bright Lime Green Trailer 120
45. Freedom (Quest for Independence) 125
46. Piano Man 129
47. Lottery 134
48. Acceptance 137
49. Reinvention 140
50. Blessing 143
51. Bulldog 146
52. Origins 151
53. Grumpy Old Fart 155
Acknowledgments 161
About the Author & Illustrator 163

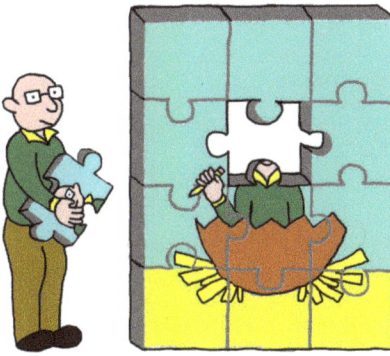

Reflections, Ramblings & Rantings of a Rancorous Stroke Survivor

FOREWORD

By: Dr. Jamila Minga, PhD., CCC-SLP. Asst. Prof. Duke University

Awareness fuels acceptance. I don't mean acceptance as in passive concession but rather awareness that aids in the ability to acknowledge each stage of stroke recovery and the resulting changes in daily living while permitting oneself and loved ones to reminisce about the old ways and grow to graciously welcome the new ways as challenging and sometimes hazardous, but nevertheless fulfilling in many respects. Awareness is challenging for most individuals after right hemisphere stroke. As a speech language pathologist and clinical researcher of communication changes, I work to improve overall awareness of the right hemisphere stroke experience. This is no easy feat as the impairment profile; particularly, related to communication is hidden from the unfamiliar and masked by relatively preserved use of sentences and words. It is, in fact, in the daily communicative interactions that insight is gained.

I've had the pleasure of developing professional and somewhat therapeutic relationships, for myself and survivors, with a number of right hemisphere stroke survivors, but none have made such a lasting impact on me as Mr. Simon Barton.

Simon and I met five years ago at a Triangle Aphasia Project (TAP) meeting where I gave a talk about right hemisphere brain damage and the resulting communication changes. After the talk, he eagerly agreed to participate in my study and shortly after his testing session stated, "Jamila darling, I feel that I need to go to the pub after that. I wouldn't do that to my worst enemy." He then followed up with a few more comments and left the lobby but returned to say, "I hope that my comments weren't off putting or offensive" to which I responded, "Simon, I like the banter." Although years post stroke, Simon's awareness was burgeoning and like most speech language pathologists who see an inkling of revelation, I pushed him to stretch a bit more and invited him to speak to my class. Simon was hesitant and not confident in his post-stroke presentation skills. With gentle encouragement, he agreed that he knew much more about his recovery than my students and that there was safety in that. Simon's presentation was phenomenal. He, emotional after the talk, expressed an appreciation for the opportunity and let me know that this was his first presentation since his stroke. I didn't know that my class talk would catapult his expressive language ventures, but I'm so pleased that it did. Changes after right hemisphere stroke have maintained a position of elusive and immeasurable and there is a dearth of information on the survivor's perspective of recovery. In this collection of poems, Simon provides a rare glimpse into the travails of the right hemisphere recovery experience—one of developing awareness. His poems highlight stereotypic characteristics of impairments while offering a view of acceptance and culminating in happiness. I often tell my students that one of the greatest gifts that we can give our patients is to listen and hear their stories. Reading Simon's perspective on recovery through creative prose is an enlightening experience and one that we as loved ones, clinicians, and physicians of right brain stroke survivors need to lend a close ear to not only for the benefit of the survivors but our own juxtaposition to recovery.

Simon, darling, I am so very grateful that our paths crossed on your journey. Keep writing good rhymes for a perfectly honorable reason.

In love, Jamila

PREFACE

It has been a while since the publication of my first effort *Not So Green as Cabbage Looking* which chronicled my early experience(s) of the Stroke I suffered along with the ups and downs associated with the recovery process. The book pretty much concluded with my eventual acceptance of the resulting deficits and despite my pursuit of the various recommended rehab therapies, the only thing I really learned (which contradicted where the book started) was that the experts were right all along and that NEVER does a brain injury/stroke affect two people the same way. I am sure for those that managed to read through to the end must have determined that in my case, I was a lost cause and unlikely to show much improvement in the future. Well, I can confirm that in many respects and without hesitation, such sentiments are absolutely, correct!

I have met with numerous, highly skilled Physical, Speech and Occupational Therapists, and despite their best efforts, they eventually came to their senses by expelling me from their various programs on the basis that I did not show the necessary willingness to work hard (particularly outside their office), and they were far better off devoting their precious hours to those that really made the effort to listen and get better. I "was not showing any functional improvement" as my most recent OT said to me as she held the door open for me to walk through. It is not that I didn't try to work at the exercise drills they all gave me but rather, after less than 10 minutes of trying and getting absolutely nothing in response, I simply gave up.

I am not sure whether my motivation to undertake the many physical drills I should be doing (at least) 4-5 times every day to help my left side limbs was taken from me by the brain injury, since pre-stroke I was a pretty determined, self-motivated sort of chap or whether my newly found interest with writing things down following the 4-5 rest breaks and daydreaming sessions I would have daily is truly the root of it all. For I must confess, I have always been a bit of a daydreamer which I do not regard as a terrible thing, after all, some of the best engineering developments I ever made as a younger man came to me on a trip somewhere to "Noddy Land".

Reflections, Ramblings & Rantings of a Rancorous Stroke Survivor

The idea for this book started with, what was supposed to be, an apology to my fabulous Occupational Therapist at the time, Cindy Wolfe OTR/L, CSRS. She designed an exercise/drill to help train my left bicep muscle and despite my very vocal huffing, puffing, moans and groans through the first set of 10 reps, she followed up by saying "good job, now let's do another 10", when all of a sudden, it just came out... "You cow!" I exclaimed, which was met with a look of disbelief along with, "what did you call me?" In an effort to save a little face I tried to convince her that the remark was not meant to be offensive but actually more of an expression of fondness, a sort of term of endearment but it was rapidly becoming clear that my powers of persuasion were falling on deaf ears, especially when other Therapists within earshot came over to console and take her side. Since I really did think the world of her, I thought I should write an apology when I got home. As a notorious Dogmatist, admitting I was wrong and saying sorry did not come naturally to me, so my token effort ended up trying to justify my position in the form of a whimsical verse (or two). I was quite pleased with my composition particularly when she smiled after reading it (although she was probably just humoring me) and as I continued to take future daybreaks, other experiences would come to mind and as the title implies, with no real connection, no rhyme nor reason, as I completed each piece, I would show it off to my wife, Sarah, when she got home from work. "Did you call the bank like I asked?" she might say, "No, but I did write this thing, what do you think?" Rolling her eyes as I gave her the piece of paper, always one for encouragement, she generally responded with some kind of sarcastic comment, "mmm, very good dear" (followed by a pause and mumbling under her breath, "... I'm sure,") - As the collection of pieces grew so did the target for book number two, 100 pages, 100 poems! This goal seemed quite doable especially as I was knocking them out sometimes at the rate of 3-4 per week. However, for someone that is not intellectually astute or literary creative, like me, I found I needed to produce around five attempts just to get one, half decent, acceptable piece! Hopefully, the selection I kept, deserve their place in this book. That, as they say, is for you to decide!

I should point out that a great number of poems did not make the final cut either because my daughter or the Publishing Editor deemed them to be too far "below the belt" (or too "un-PC"!) Of the few I managed to sneak in, I really am sorry if you are offended, but I didn't produce this thing to be liked and/or to limit the audience to a particularly like-minded select group.

As you will see (should you get that far), my approach to my post stroke (recovery) journey evolved more into a journey of discovery which turned into a quest to redefine myself, a journey of reinvention, and a journey with no end. But then, all of us, regardless of circumstance, have our life's courses to run. I worry sometimes, that the day before I take my last breath, I will still be concerned and wondering what I can do to place a positive spin on my life since that rotten event back in May 2013, how I can make it better for me, and those close to me. How and can one ever stop? If I ever get to answer that question, it might serve as an interesting subject matter for book number three!

I can only hope that you are reasonably open-minded and can forgive me all my many sins along the way! Please also note these reflections are not in any particular order, again, for no rhyme nor reason. Should you find the occasional theme or inference a little offensive, my conscience is clear, because I did warn you ahead of time. You proceed at your own risk!

1. ASPIRING POET

I have always enjoyed the process of writing, not that I have ever been very good at it. My earliest schoolboy memories take me back to the numerous times I was kept after lessons and made to write a hundred times, sentences like, "I must not talk in class, I must not talk …" etc., etc.

That said, and despite the formal education I was lucky enough to receive, I consistently failed the mandatory English Literature exams we were obliged to take to move onward and upward. After graduating engineering college and a short spell doing a toolmaking apprenticeship, I went to work for my father, a man who was a very gifted writer. I took the opportunity and benefitted from his regular critiques of the many business documents I was obliged to write, through which, I learned a great deal. Up until my mid-twenties, most of my writing was limited to technical documents like manuals, sales brochures, formal quotations and covering letters and only as I ventured into the area of marketing did any kind of creativity begin to creep in. Future job responsibilities expanded my needs as I took on more senior roles and so my business writing skills needed to expand accordingly. Conference papers and business plans were becoming a regular thing, and I began to enjoy the satisfaction gained from completing each assignment.

Following the stroke, my first (outpatient) SLP, Maura English Silverman. MS, CCC/SLP, made it her mission to encourage me to, "write as much as possible" to at least, "be sure to maintain a daily journal" and when I would have something on my mind, "write yourself a little essay about it and we can discuss it later together". Through her weekly encouragement, every opportunity I had (when I was not napping) I would write something. As with all strokes, not only does the survivor lose some physical skills but cognitive ones as well; one thing I did not lose (sadly), was the ability to stick my big mouth in places where it was not welcome. I dread to think how many letters of apology I wrote over those first couple of years following the stroke event. But there is a good chance that if you had the misfortune to have provided me some kind of post stroke therapy, you will have likely received a letter of apology on those occasions; my tongue was ahead of my brain. I remember in one of Maura's group lessons when she had each of us read a paragraph of an article associated with stroke recovery, and after my turn, she said, "I do like the way you speak Simon, just the way you just said the word, 'grass'" [emphasizing my pronunciation, "Grarse"]. I quickly quipped, "Funny you should say that Maura, I wonder has anyone told you that you have a lovely Arse?" On the one hand, it got a chuckle from the group, but on the other, if looks could kill… Definitely an opportunity to write, yet another, letter of apology!

I have never been a fast learner; it takes a while for me to be schooled on anything, it seems to take forever for any message to fully sink in and that fact haunts me to this day. I was warned by my first (rehab) SLP to be careful with my language since the stroke event had probably caused a loss "to [my] filters", and "you will be prone to saying things you might regret!" she said. Clearly, I didn't learn from that excellent advice.

Despite the extensive practice I have had over the years and particularly more recently, it will not take you long to determine that I have never fully mastered the art of classical verse. I can appreciate the quality of works of notable poets like Shakespeare, Wordsworth, and Blake and the American, Edgar Allan Poe, but not to the extent that I have the first idea as to how they went about the creation process. I certainly do not have their talents nor their extraordinary (and sometimes, abstract) vocabulary to draw upon. So, this, my first poem, I hoped, might set the tone for the rest. I think it portrays the limited literary style and quality that follows, (sorry).

With that said, now might be a good time for you to file the book on the "Give to Charity" shelf or wrap it up for next year's Christmas present to give to your least favorite relative (even better if they happen to be like me, "mentally challenged!")

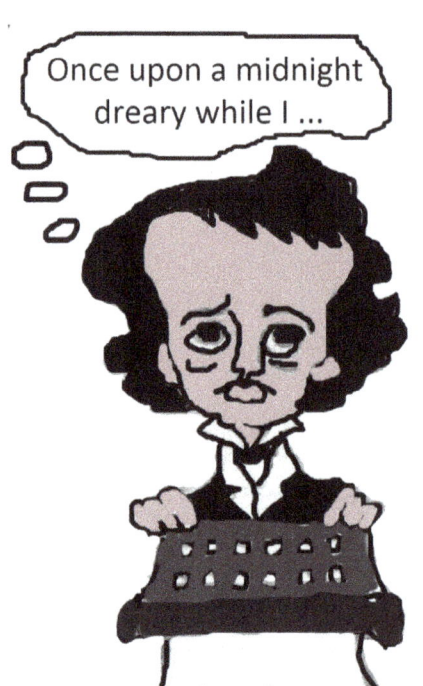
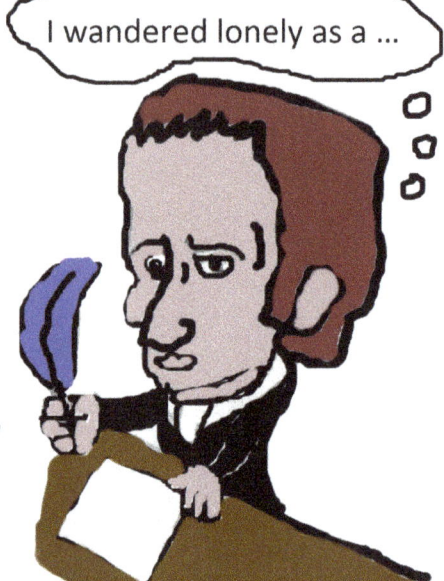

ASPIRING POET

With limited mobility I had to do something,
Moping around was quite unbecoming,
One silly rhyme was all that it took,
When someone proposed I should place in a book,
I will never aspire to Wordsworth or Poe,
But you have to start somewhere, why not give it a go?

I have found it tough to get in my say,
When writing has helped much more to convey,
My feelings might take a while to create,
But, with no interruptions, no time for debate…

I pour out my thoughts then re-read the words,
Delete as I need and modify verbs,
Keep making changes until it is ratified,
And won't stop the process until I am satisfied,
That's not to say, it's like Wordsworth or Poe,
But it's the best I can do, with the words that I know,

The content of few may be hostile, tough to embrace,
The intent was to pursue a small smile to your face.

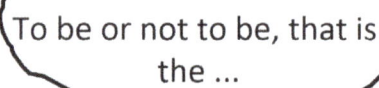
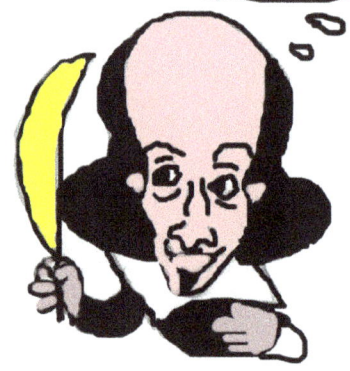
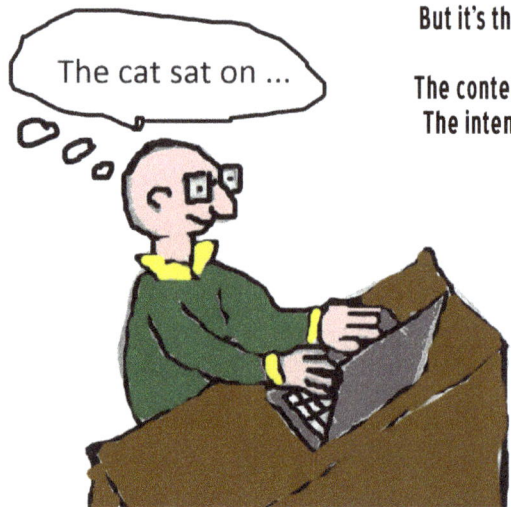

2. SIMON'S STORY

It is only proper that if I am to use the vehicle of writing as some kind of excuse to make mockery of something or somebody then at the very least, I must fess up about my own failings.

I owned and managed my own company, an engineering design and manufacturing business. We were doing very well; sales were good with a strong order book that bode well for the future. We had just developed a new technology that was in the process of obtaining a worldwide patent. I was working crazy hours to keep up. As with many small businesses expanding too quickly, cash was short and any feelings of joy and excitement about the future were countered by even stronger feelings of concern and worry about our financial wellbeing. I was under a lot of stress and did not know which way to turn.

I played a competitive game of tennis every Thursday evening and as I struggled to get my breath during a tough rally, I tended to blame my advancing years before even considering the all-too-frequent alcoholic drink and smoke I habitually had the moment I got home from work.

The writing (I didn't read), was well and truly on the wall and it was only a matter of time that I would experience a life changing medical event.

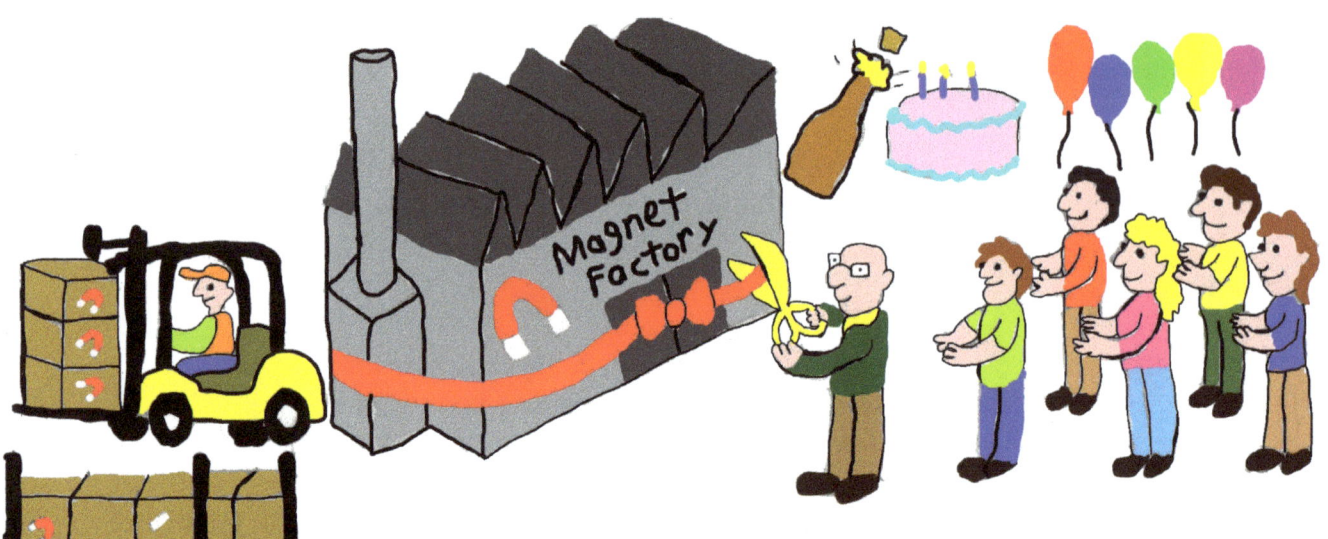

SIMON'S STORY

There was this middle-aged bloke,
Who liked to drink and to smoke,

He had to admit,
He worked like a twit,

Eventually rushed off with a stroke!

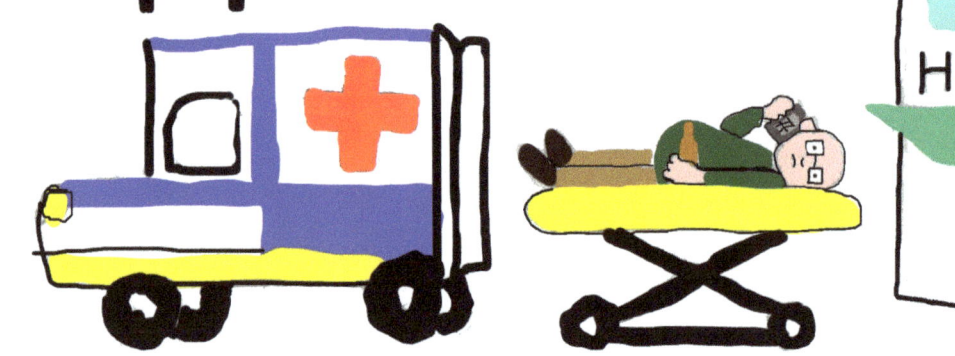

3. THE JOURNEY

I spent one (long) week in the ICU ward of the hospital when I was first admitted. Once I had "stabilized" I was referred and transferred to a well-regarded (local) hospital that specialized in stroke rehab.

Without exception, all the medical professionals assigned to me during those first few weeks, made it brutally clear that the process of recovery was not going to be short and easy but more likely, long and arduous—certainly, nobody made any promises. But when I left there a few months later, I had enough strength and coordination to stand and make it more feasible for Sarah (benefitting from her own lessons), to transfer me from a wheelchair to the car and vice-versa or chair to bed, wheelchair to the couch and so on. I was capable enough to go home and had advanced to a level that my journey of recovery could continue with outpatient therapies— or so I thought.

Although I was thrilled to be home, it was not as straightforward as we thought. We lived in a two-story house and the bedroom was upstairs. Fortunately, Luke our second son, was at home and with his strength, between them, they managed to drag me up there each evening, somehow. I had to keep a bedpan on my bedside table so that I didn't have to wake Sarah in the middle of the night in order for her to wheel me to the bathroom and set me on the loo.

It has been (and will continue to be) a journey with no rules of the road; heck, not even a road map to follow, so best we just keep trudging along, I guess.

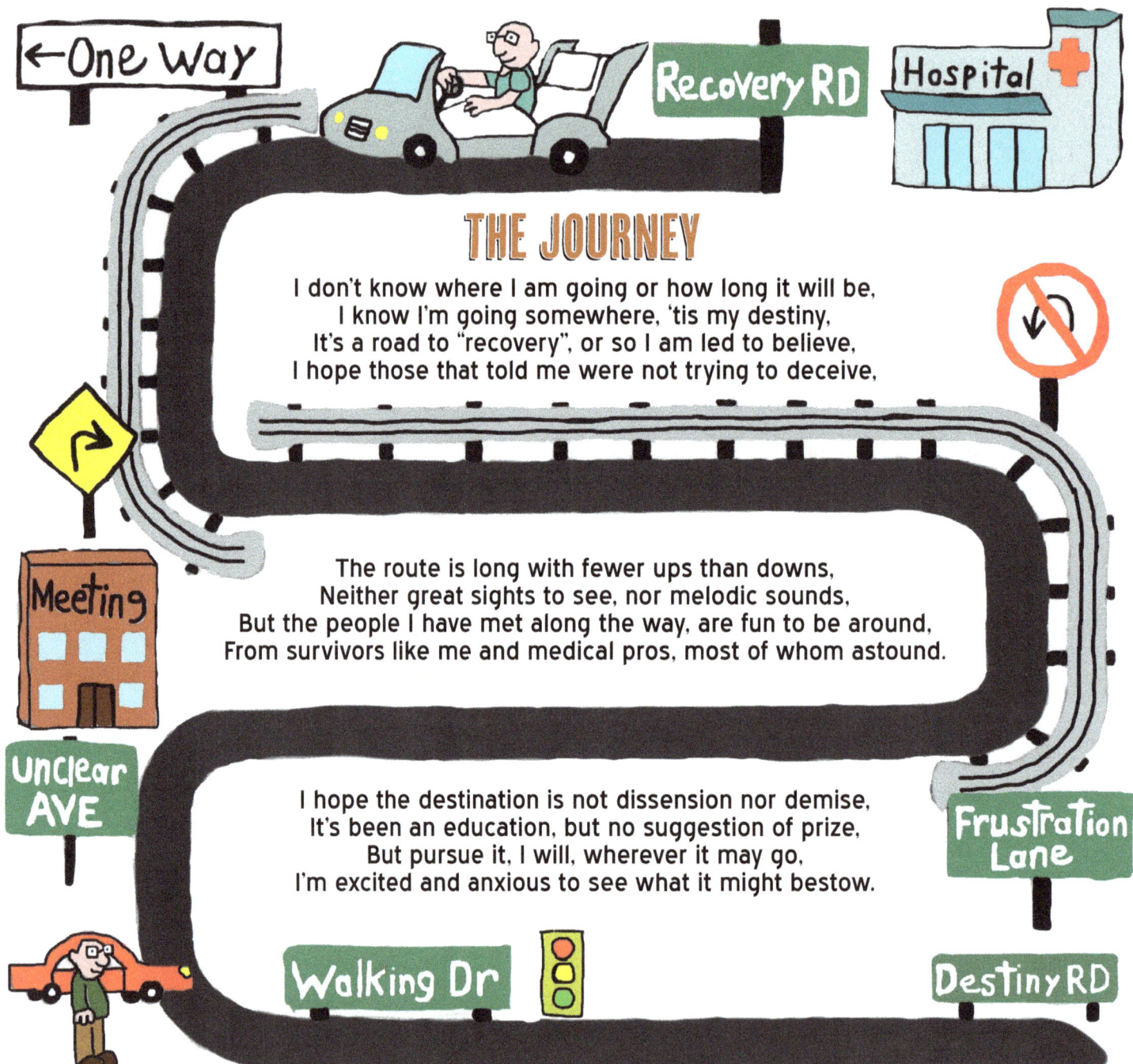

4. ANGELS

Everyone knows the value and importance the Nurse plays within our healthcare systems, but I contend that it is only when you or a loved-one is confined to a hospital bed and in need of 24-hour care can you truly appreciate the dedication and professionalism displayed by these heroes in uniform. I spent 36 hours in the ICU department before being transferred to the Rehab hospital where I would then be labeled a "fall-risk" which meant even more one to one time as the nurse maneuvered me from bed to wheelchair and back again. My ongoing cardiology issues would mean more hospital visits and more encounters with Nurses.

My last heart ablation procedure (two years ago) did not go to plan and involved an overnight stay at the hospital. I sincerely felt that from that point onward, the nurse would be spared Simon for some time (famous last words) …

Recently, I volunteered to drive my friend, Ronald, to and from a local hospital so that he could undergo a surgical procedure – it wasn't terribly major, but with the anesthetics involved, the doctor emphasized the need for some support. As usual, I underestimated the waiting time and found myself wandering the seemingly endless floors and corridors to find somewhere to eat. Typically, the first (and nearest) cafeteria was closed and the alternative establishment, had to be the furthest distance from Ronald's ward. At the "speed of Simon" it took me ages to find the place. By the time I eventually arrived, I really worked up an appetite and quickly got in line for the special of the day, "Shrimp and Grits". The convenience of walking with a cane soon became a major inconvenience when considering the need to carry a polystyrene box of food and a bottle of coke, particularly when you cannot use your other hand to help! I was definitely the bottleneck that day - I'm sure the majority of Nurses and Doctors that were behind me were regretting they did not take the opportunity to drive off-site to the more expensive restaurant down the road that day! When I finally arrived at the checkout, I realized that I stupidly left my wallet in the car - about a mile away!! Sheepishly, I placed my box on the counter and apologized profusely to the cashier that I did not have the funds with me to pay but would return shortly and headed for the exit. I had not got very far when a lady in a white uniform caught up with me and said, "excuse me Sir, please let me pay for your meal." This Nurse had obviously followed me around and overheard my exchange with the Cashier, I was a little overcome and started to cry and before I could protest, she had picked up my food and presented the bar code on her identity pass to the scanner and the transaction was done. "Now where are you sitting?" she said as she escorted me to an empty table. Within a couple of seconds after sitting down, another Nurse came over to me with some cutlery and a napkin, "you might need these," she said and then another Nurse came over and asked, "can I undo the cap on your coke bottle for you?" Nurses seemed to be coming out of the woodwork, Nurses everywhere!

My moist eyes did not clear for the whole time I wolfed down my food which I ate in double-quick time.

It is not difficult to conclude that the Nurse was simply "born to be". I refuse to accept that the level of compassion, caring and empathy required for the profession is solely a result of the multitude of rigorous training programs necessary for qualification.

I have had (and continue to have) more than my fair share of Nurses, sadly for them, they have had (and continue to have) more than their fair share of me!

With all that said, here is my small thank you and tribute...

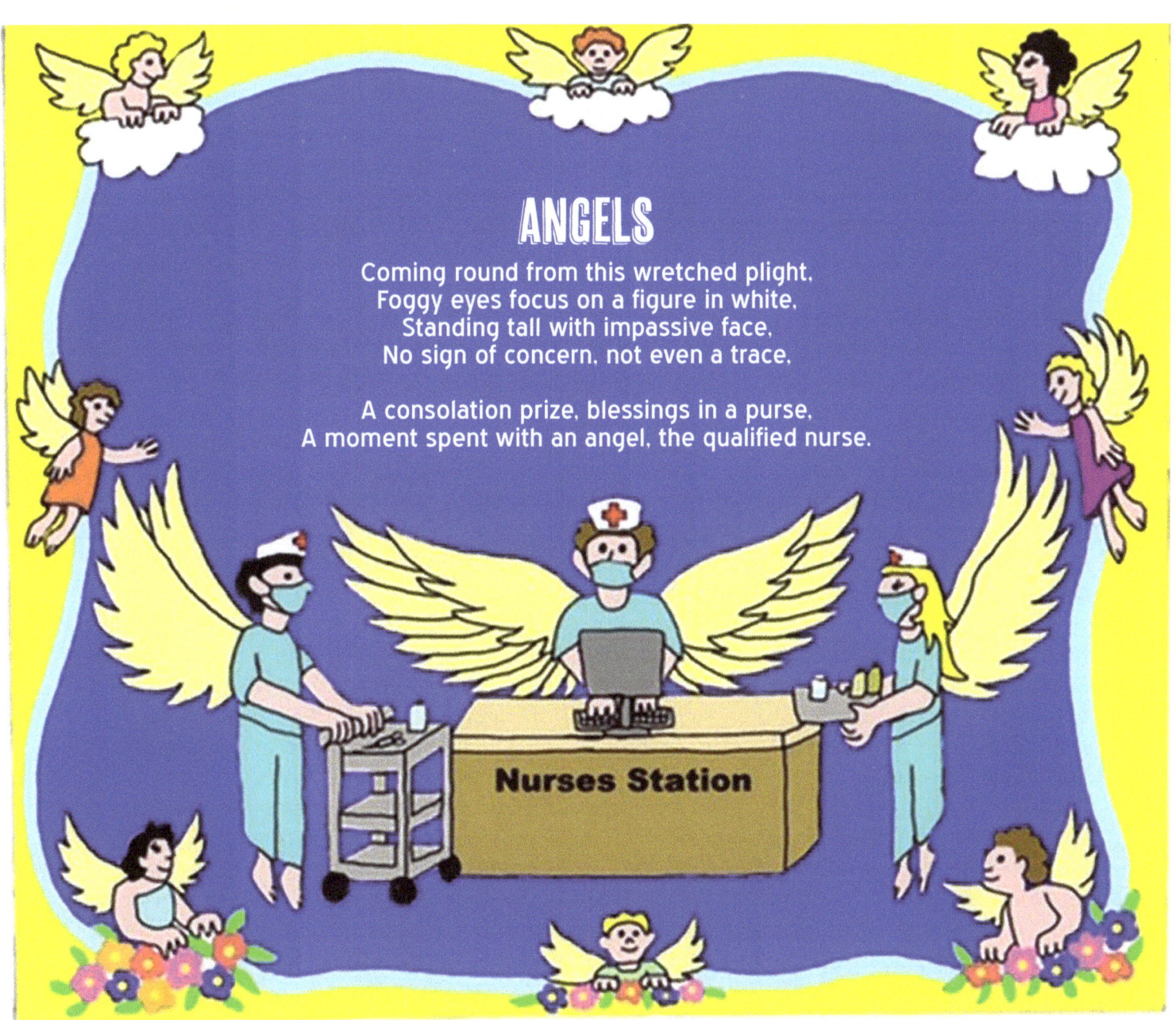

5. THE THERAPIST

It has been over six years since I was released from rehab hospital where I would commence my stroke recovery journey proper. At the time of departure, I was armed with a list of highly recommended (local) outpatient clinics to continue my treatment within the areas of speech, occupational and physical therapies—all necessary to help progress me through the next few years.

Following a recent review, I determined that during this time, I had met and received treatment from at least, seventeen different professionals and without exception, all were extremely talented, and all have contributed positively to my journey and future well-being.

I found that going to therapy for a stroke survivor is a bit like going to school for a child—having lost many of those abilities that as infants, we simply learned naturally by trial and error—we now have to learn it all again but with a more focused approach in the interest of safety and simply doing it the right way; once the therapist teaches us the technique we must then do homework to practice and perfect it.

My career would suggest someone that must have been well educated backed up with impressive qualifications, but the truth of the matter is that I scraped by my school years and for the most part, was lucky to be in the right place at the right time on more than one occasion. I managed to fool my way through those important career opportunities. Somehow, the immigration lawyer that was hired to handle my work transfer from England to my new employer here in North Carolina managed to persuade the United States Government that I was worthy of an EB-1 Visa a "Person of Extraordinary Ability"! A work-visa that is usually reserved for top scientists in some kind of critical field of medical research, for example; or you might be entitled to one if you happen to be one of the world's top athletes with a potential to represent the US at the next Olympics. I must say, I felt a little guilty and quite embarrassed when that certificate came through the mail one day.

As a student, I was too busy daydreaming to pay attention to the teacher; the occasions I did take notice were generally limited to those times I was being disciplined for being disrespectful or downright rude. It is no wonder that as I write this chapter, I have no therapy sessions lined up having been expelled from most of them. Just before my mother died, I said to her local parish vicar when she was in earshot, "well, you know Nick, I was expelled from more schools than I graduated," and being typically proud, prim and proper, Mum, clearly vexed by my comment, cut in with, "you were not expelled … you were asked to leave! [Err, a couple of times]."

Despite the fact that my past therapists are probably pleased to not have me back—I would not have me back—their skills and time should be reserved to those that need it most and follow their instructions diligently. Above all, I recognize that it was through their efforts that I am mobile and function to the extent that, not only could Sarah go out to work, but when she got home, I was still alive and the house had not burned down!

It is only right, therefore, that I give a little tribute to these (all too often) unsung heroes in scrubs!

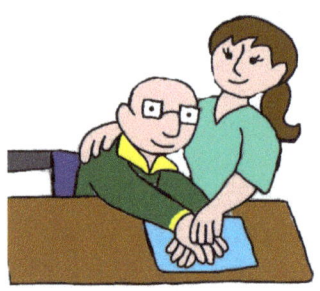
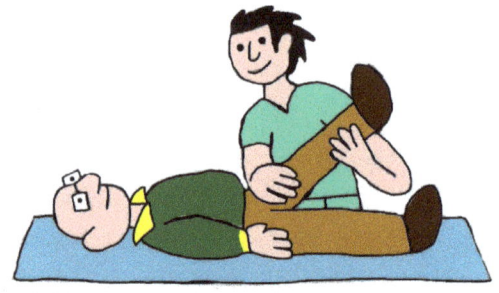
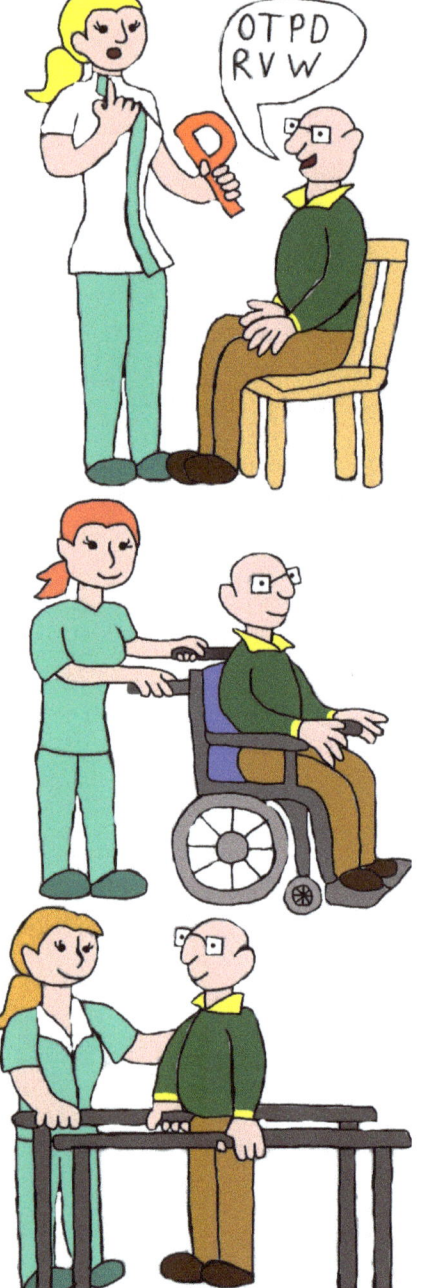

THE THERAPIST

The professional Therapist is something to behold,
Loads of experience but seldom old,
Doctors without the title, but "great as", in my eyes,
Paid much less, it just ain't right!

The skills possessed and the support they deliver,
Make them the ultimate Caregiver,

I love my SLP, PT and OT,
And wish I could take them all home with me,

The highlight of the week is Therapy Day,
Second only to when I hear one say,
"Good job today, you are on your way!"

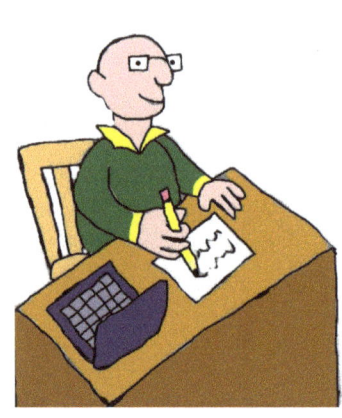
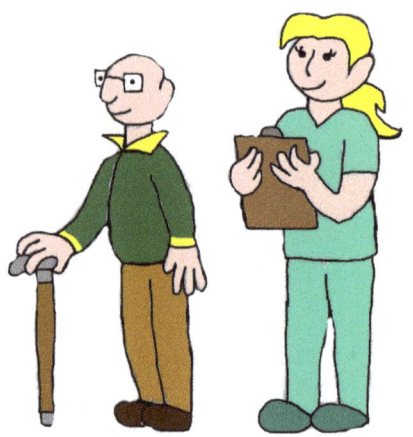

BAD RHYMES, NO REASON

6. APHASIA

The brain injury I received was caused by a simple "blockage" of blood supply—a blood clot lodged itself in an artery and cut off the supply of much needed oxygen (within the blood) (this type of stroke is known as "ischemic") and was located to an area at the middle cerebral artery to the right hemisphere/side of the brain and whilst it impacted me physically to my left side limbs, my communicative skills were much less impacted than those unfortunate survivors that suffered a brain injury to the left hemisphere—particularly the left frontal lobe region (also known as "Broca's area") since these injuries typically result with significant limitations to speaking and listening as well as reading and writing—the very definition of "aphasia". That said, I still required the professional assistance of a speech language pathologist (SLP) to help me manage some organizational and slightly lesser communication issues.

My (out-patient) SLP encouraged me to join a local charity group called "Triangle Aphasia Project" (TAP) headquartered in Cary, North Carolina. This put me in touch with other stroke survivors and to this day, I continue to marvel and be inspired by their efforts to address both their physical and communicative weaknesses. I wanted to take the opportunity to reference this excellent organization within this book, first, in the hope you might like to donate toward the tremendous work they do and second, to promote the word "aphasia" since very few people outside the stroke survivor and neuro-medical has ever heard the term. Indeed, a recent national survey suggested that despite there being over 2 million aphasia sufferers in the US alone, around 86 percent of the population has no idea what aphasia means as a medical condition, I certainly didn't – do you?

Aphasia is the loss of ability to understand or express speech resulting from a brain injury.

"Imagine…" as TAP promotes, "…the last word you said was the last word you said… Period!"

I would like to point out, that aphasia, as experienced by a left-hemisphere, brain-injury as many stroke survivors have received, resulting from an interruption of blood supply to the brain (ischemic or hemorrhagic) is a treatable condition which largely through the talent and skills of a qualified SLP, often show positive (restorative) results. There is a condition known as primary progressive aphasia (PPA) which whilst treatable, as the name suggests, can progressively worsen and full communicative skills are harder to restore.

Lastly, people with aphasia are cognitively intact (non-linguistically), executive functioning and memory, for example, are not unduly affected—it is purely a language disorder (memory and executive functioning are not generally related). I continue to have quite deep, meaningful and intellectual conversations with a left-brain stroke survivor, in those first couple of years post the actual stroke event—it may be that we need to be a little more patient and understanding as the stroke survivor sometimes has to fight to find that word or a roundabout way to deliver their message, but cognitively and in many respects, they are quite sharp.

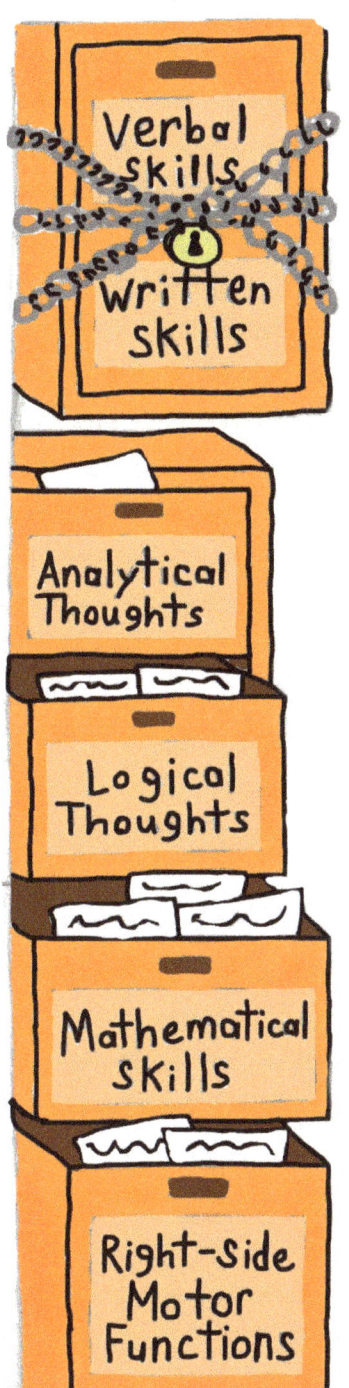
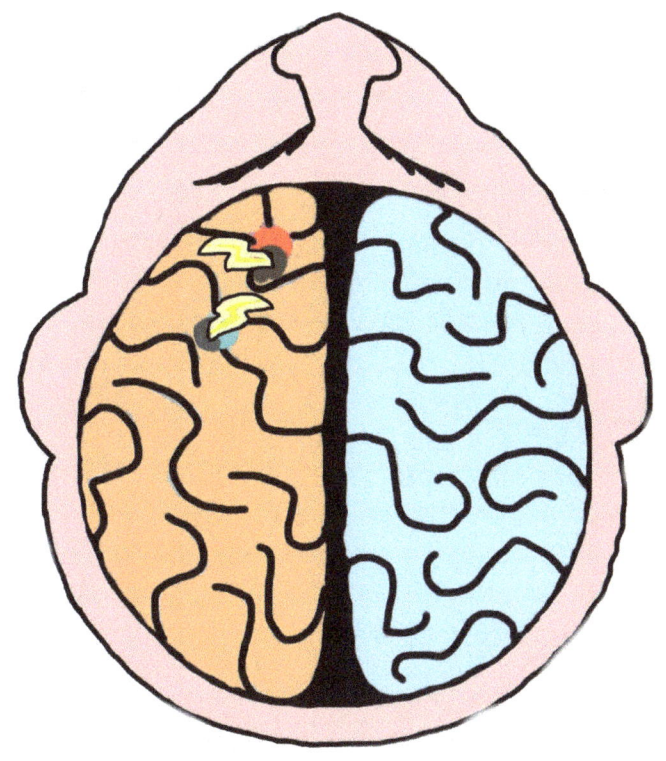
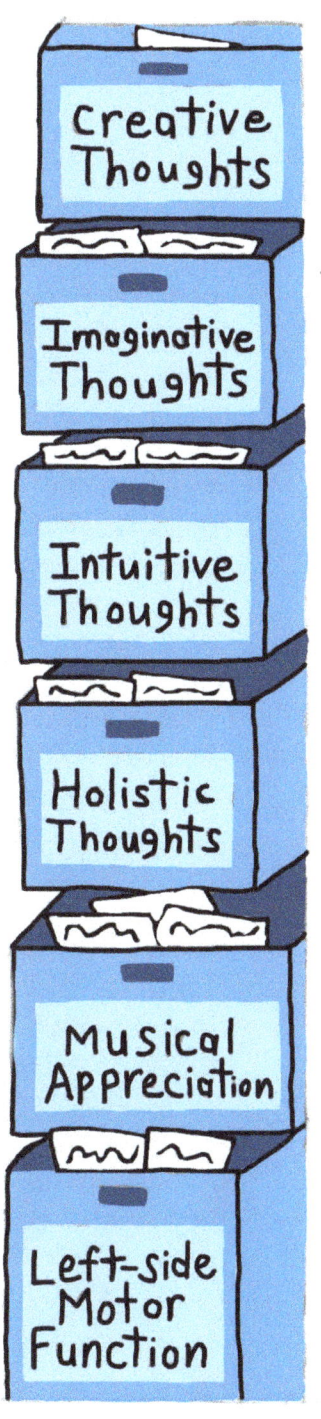

APHASIA

'Twas lucky the brain injury was to my right,
Causing Hemiparesis and some issues with sight,
But normalcy, whilst challenging was still within reach,
I had not the burden of losing my speech,

Those less blessed with damage to the left,
Have communication abilities, bereft,

But with love, care and specialist assistance,
Lots of patience and tons of perseverance,

The speech that they yearn,
Will, one day, return.

Reflections, Ramblings & Rantings of a Rancorous Stroke Survivor

7. HEAVEN AND HELL

Thanks to my stroke along with my inability to hold a typical 9-5 job away from home, I have way too much time on my hands, to relax, reflect and reminisce on areas of my life where I have experienced both good and bad things and how external influences have affected our family and shaped me as a person, my character and some of my political viewpoints. It was during one of those quiet ruminations that I remembered an old joke I was told as a young businessman starting my second job for an Italian company and it occurred to me that I could keep its structure but make up my own variation and put it to verse. Recent events have caused me to become more of an "anti-globalist" these days, but I have had the good fortune to travel much of the world and see, first-hand, both the positives and negatives behind the many countries I visited; their cultures and the unique character of their people and where they stand in the world. Being the weird guy that I am, it was only natural I would come up with the following iteration.

On a more serious note, I don't think it would be a stretch to see it as a metaphor of what life can seem like when someone like me (now that I have been in the "recovery" phase for a while) contrasts their life "before a stroke" with their life "after a stroke"—things can appear a bit out of sorts—a definite and similar sort of contradiction exists … pre-stroke I was, highly ambitious, working up to 80 (crazy) hours per week thinking I could retire with a successful business under my belt having made a sizeable lump of money to shore up a financially secure retirement for the years to come. In addition, I still managed to fit in some serious play time, tennis and golf particularly, and would never miss the opportunity of a good old booze up with close friend. whereas poststroke, I have seriously mellowed to become more content with a 15-20 hour (maximum) work week and reserve my social activity to a weekend afternoon with family and maybe, if we are feeling particularly naughty, my wife and I could stretch to an evening cocktail on one of her days off! Physically I go for a 20-minute walk (at the speed of Simon) each morning, and I am quite happy to leave tennis and golf for others to pursue—It's quite enough effort for me to get up from my recliner to get the remote control and watch it on the telly, thank you.

Forgive me for the fact there is a fair amount of stereotyping associated with some of the portrayals depicted in the piece, but I hope you can appreciate the various ironies behind the message.

Considering the vast background and heritage associated with the different nationalities referenced, there should be at least two lines that each reader will glean a little satisfaction and frustration in equal measure; if I got it right that is; but then you will be the judge of that, I am sure!

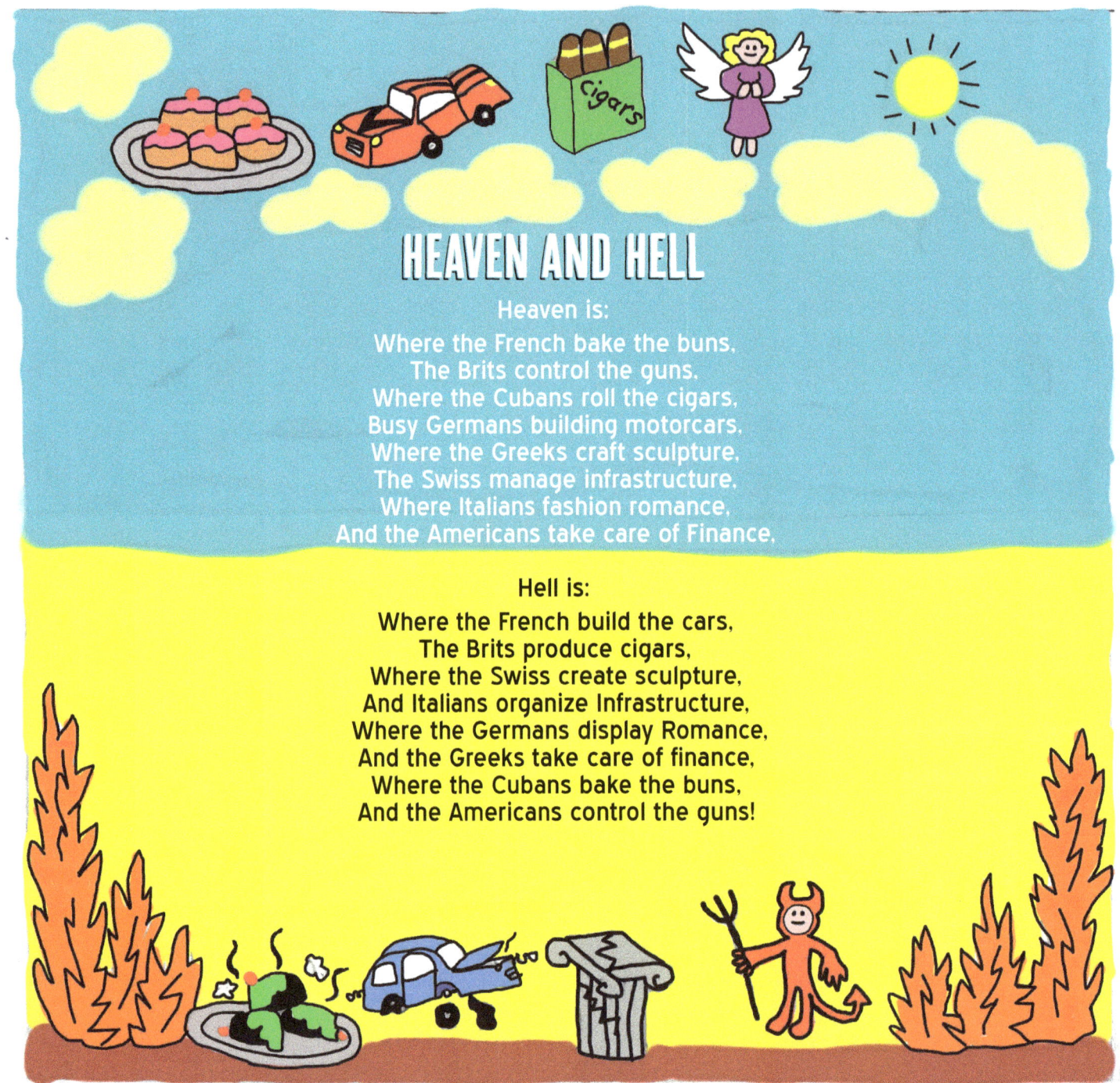

HEAVEN AND HELL

Heaven is:

Where the French bake the buns,
The Brits control the guns.
Where the Cubans roll the cigars,
Busy Germans building motorcars.
Where the Greeks craft sculpture,
The Swiss manage infrastructure.
Where Italians fashion romance,
And the Americans take care of Finance.

Hell is:

Where the French build the cars,
The Brits produce cigars,
Where the Swiss create sculpture,
And Italians organize Infrastructure,
Where the Germans display Romance,
And the Greeks take care of finance,
Where the Cubans bake the buns,
And the Americans control the guns!

8. TERM OF ENDEARMENT

As referenced in the preface, this next poem was the initial motivation behind this book and was meant to be an apology for calling my occupational therapist, Cindy, a "cow" when I felt she was driving me too hard one day. As you will see, the so-called apology was not unequivocal and ended up more of a defense/justification piece.

As a young boy growing up in England, it was not uncommon to call your sister or girlfriend a "cow" for something quite trivial and very rarely was the comment received offensively (although in both cases, my sister and girlfriend [and later my wife], did deliver me a good "whack"). I certainly do not remember my parents ever disciplining me for using the term (so maybe it is their fault). Generally speaking, I think it fair to say that calling someone a cow was reasonably limited and accepted to people you are close with; my error here is presuming such familiarity with my OT which, with the benefit of hindsight, was clearly an overestimation on my part along with the potential mismatch of cultures.

Since moving to North Carolina thirty years ago, I am no stranger to saying the wrong thing at the wrong time. As George Bernard Shaw observed, "England and America are separated by a common language". An example of my many misjudgments can be seen when I said to a group of factory workers, after the sounding of the tea break bell: "just in time, as it happens, I would love a fag right now!" (They did not know that a "fag" to me was a slang term for a cigarette and at the time, I certainly did not know what a "fag" meant to them). Then there was the time, when following a drawing error, I went to my newly appointed lady secretary and asked whether she might have a rubber I could use. After the inevitable, "what sort of woman do you take me for?" type comments and the ensuing quite disagreeable discussion, we finally worked out that a "rubber" in England is known as an "eraser" in America, and I was eventually forgiven that day although the same secretary had the audacity to say to me one afternoon, I have typed your letters and corrected all your spelling mistakes—where did you learn your English!?". "You Cow", I thought but didn't say out loud (because I didn't like her very much).

When recuperating in rehab hospital, the resident speech language pathologist warned me "to be careful because you have likely lost all your filters". This was probably one of the worst things a medical professional could say to me. In her defense, she was not to know that I had very few filters to begin with, but now she has given me a medical excuse to say whatever was on my mind. Those first three or four poststroke years had me writing letters of apologies at the rate of two or three per month, due to one derogatory remark, a joke in poor taste or another! Nowadays, I find it easier when meeting people for the first time to apologize in advance for the potential of being overly frank or downright rude, "because I have this medical condition, sorry."

On the one hand, speaking with a (Queen's English) accent allowed me to take a few liberties—especially when I did not have many filters pre stroke. One of my sales managers sitting in an audience during one of my lectures commented, "Simon you are so lucky, had I delivered the same spiel as you just did, I would have been thrown out the room with my feet not touching the ground! But when you used the F-word (on more than one occasion) I could see others in the audience smiling and twittering to each other, 'isn't it quaint, so sweet' and totally accepting of you." On the other hand, I am convinced that this intelligent persona/illusion had the opposite and negative effect on the numerous SLP's I would later meet as I embarked on my poststroke journey giving them the illusion that I was better than I really was. Only at some point after my time in hospital did my outpatient SLP recognize that I had many issues to contend with, which were not limited to filter less comments; clearly, I have much to learn, not unlike all my resulting ailments, I have come to accept that as far as my communication shortfalls are concerned, it is just "work in progress," and do my best to be better!

TERM OF ENDEARMENT

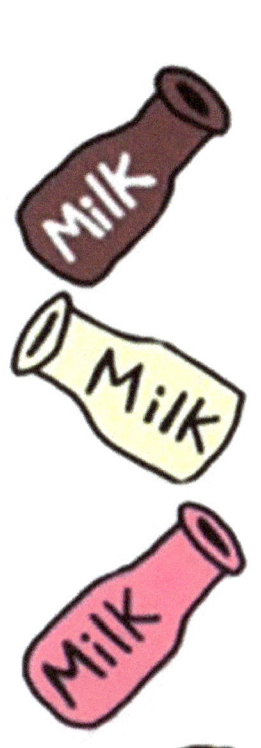

Calling you a "cow" was not said to be rude,
There was no adjective before, to make it so crude,

A "*fat cow*" or an "*ugly cow*" is a different matter,
But a *nondescript cow* was offered to flatter,

The cow is a magnificent beast,
She gives much of herself for us to feast,

To be compared with such a noble animal,
Makes my respect for you even more palpable,

So now that you have read this, I hope it is clear then,
To be called a "cow" *is*, a term of endearment.

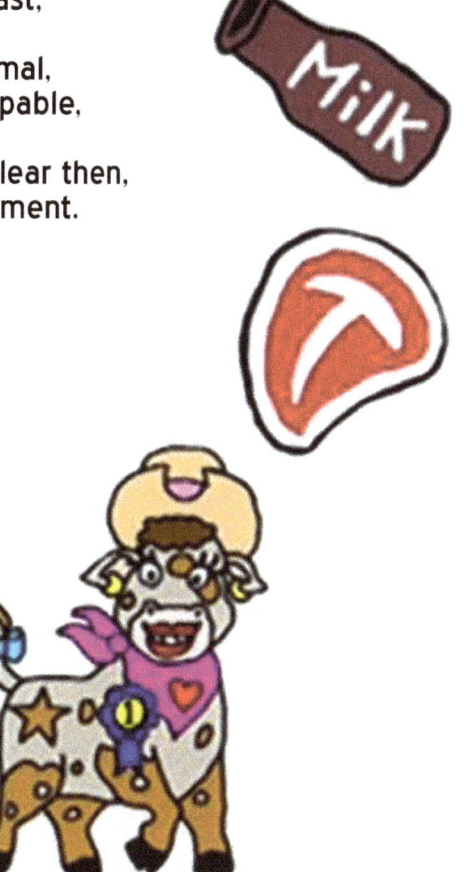

9. WHAT'S YOUR NAME AGAIN?

Memory loss is quite common following a brain injury, particularly for those of us that are no longer as young as we would like to be. My long-term memory seems to work pretty well, but I have not completely escaped some short-term memory issues either. A typical example would be coming out of my office for a coffee break only to be greeted by my wife saying, "Can you write in Samantha's birthday card, I left it on the kitchen table for you to fill out and then I can get it in the mailbox?" Getting to the table, I find there is no pen, but I have one in the office, so, I walk back to get one. Along the way, I am thinking I will also need my reading glasses and my mobile phone which I use to hold the card down as I write since it is hard for me to use my other hand. When I get to the office, I pick up the phone and make the journey back to the kitchen and only when I get back to the table do I remember (again), the pen, and start my way back to the office repeating the process only to find that only when I am sitting down, pen in hand, phone laying down the card, when I realize, I need my reading glasses and so off to the office I venture once more. At least I benefit from the exercise!

I have had the great fortune to meet many others like me, people who have survived a brain injury/stroke but to some extent, have had to deal with other, quite different issues which they battle, accommodate and through some form of reinvention, learn to live with. My friend David had a stroke whilst undergoing an open-heart surgery procedure (literally on the operating table). He suffers from the same genetic condition I have, namely, "hypertrophic cardiomyopathy." Our post event symptoms are similar but for him, it did not cause too many physical weaknesses, but unlike me, it did leave him with some aphasia and seriously compromised his executive function skills. Most impacted was his short-term memory.

David was a highly regarded and sought-after systems administrator and used to pride himself on his ability to access and recall quite complex lines of code at will, but since his stroke, he requires frequent visits to various reference manuals to help obtain the necessary information in order to undertake his work competently.

Still, he puts on a brave face, and constantly exudes a cheery disposition, making valuable contributions and advice at group meetings to the rest of us (fellow survivors) around him. And he has since adopted a warm smile on those occasions he loses track mid-sentence and obliged to ask, "I'm sorry, remind me the question you asked again?"

I have no doubt the vast improvements he has made that I have witnessed over the past few years with his overall confidence and speaking fluency will show similar gains with the memory struggles he faces today.

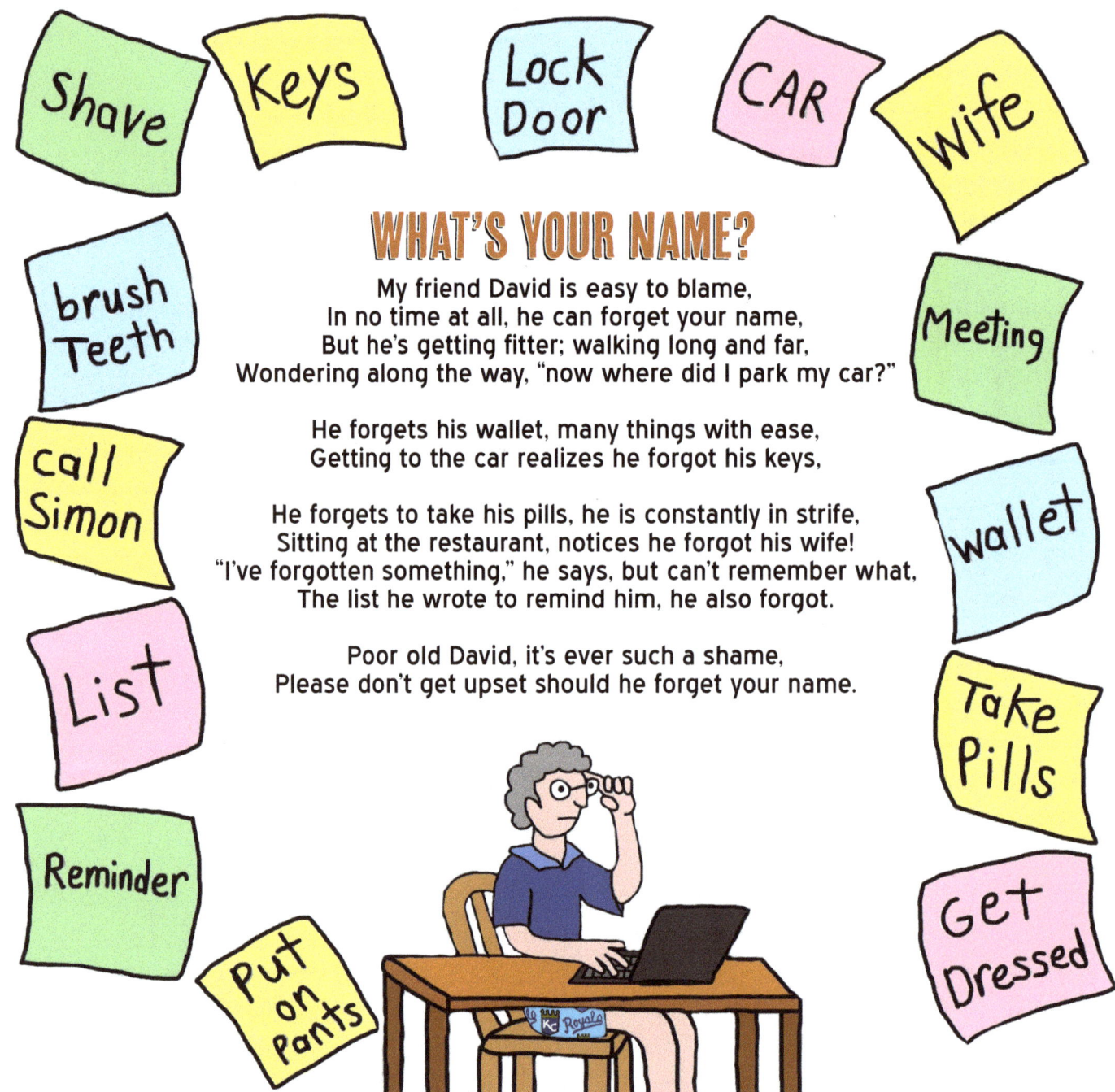

WHAT'S YOUR NAME?

My friend David is easy to blame,
In no time at all, he can forget your name,
But he's getting fitter; walking long and far,
Wondering along the way, "now where did I park my car?"

He forgets his wallet, many things with ease,
Getting to the car realizes he forgot his keys,

He forgets to take his pills, he is constantly in strife,
Sitting at the restaurant, notices he forgot his wife!
"I've forgotten something," he says, but can't remember what,
The list he wrote to remind him, he also forgot.

Poor old David, it's ever such a shame,
Please don't get upset should he forget your name.

10. AHEAD OF MY TIME

I struggle terribly with the simplest organizational tasks and in particular, the whole area of time management.

It took me forever to appreciate that those jobs I could knock out in 5 minutes pre stroke are seldom achievable in 30 minutes, post. Along with my inability to ward off distraction, it all had the inevitable result of me running late for appointments or time sensitive tasks. A typical example would be a therapy appointment to arrive in a couple of hours—loads of time, right? Enough time for me to complete that letter and get it in the mailbox before I leave? Wrong! Every last-minute task always took much longer than anticipated and all of a sudden, my appointment was now in only 30 minutes, and it is still a 20 minute drive. This unforeseen situation would cause me to panic and hurry and rushing meant making mistakes which not only makes me look foolish but just adds to the anxiety; like forgetting to take my wallet or my phone and/or the therapy aid I promised to return. It is made worse by the fact that I can no longer drive quickly and safely. In actual fact, for me, the consequence of being anxious while driving would often involve making wrong turns which only made me even later and more upset.

A couple of years of being late for appointments feeling frustrated and embarrassed has had the reverse effect, to the extent of being obsessively neurotic about it that it is almost funny how early I am now for many deadlines, as portrayed in the following verse, which, by the way, is not an exaggeration!

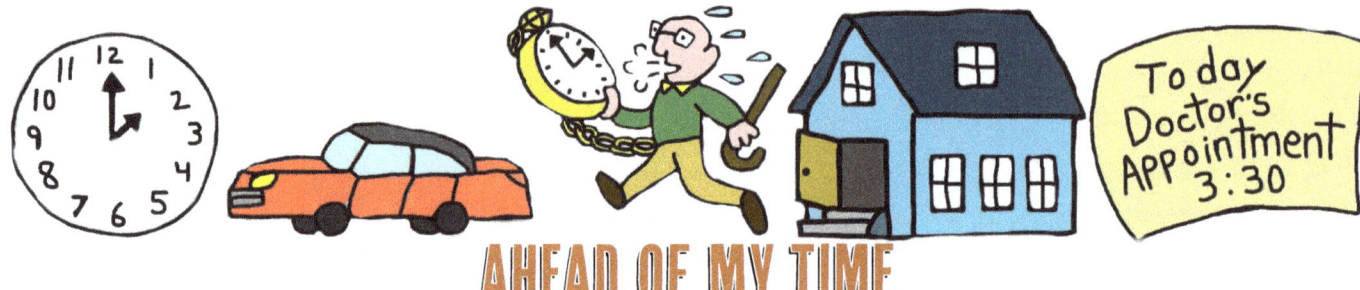

AHEAD OF MY TIME

I must see the specialist at HALF PAST THREE,
Mustn't be late; with plenty of time I should leave,

The drive should take just twenty minutes to do,
Allowing for traffic, I will leave at TWO.

The check-in process can be long and troublesome.
On second thoughts, leave closer to ONE.

Must top up my gas along the way,
So, be in the car around MIDDAY,

Forgot my wallet once and learned the lesson...
Not to rush again, depart closer to ELEVEN.

Much too early to eat before then,
Pick up a snack along the way and go at TEN.

Forgetting to stop and it was a traffic free journey,
Arriving hungry, of course, and nearly THREE HOURS EARLY!

Niggling considerations that go through my mind,
Signaling justifications for being ahead of my time!

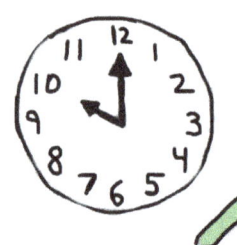
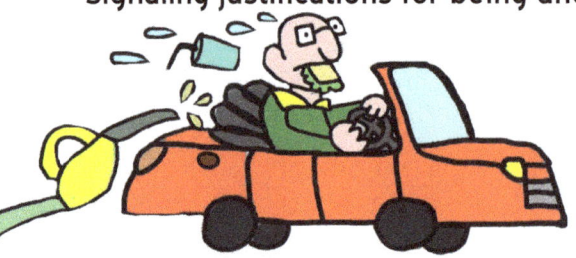
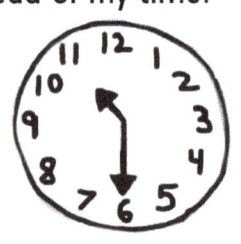
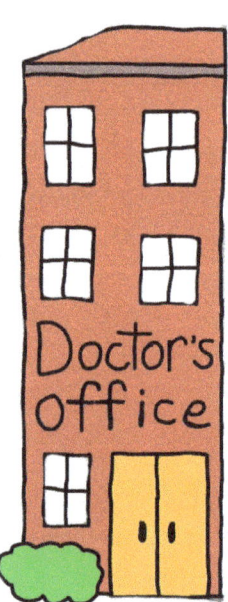

BAD RHYMES, NO REASON

11. RETICENCE

I was never the shy, quiet one that sat at the back of the class I always had something to say and regrettably, saying too much would usually get me into trouble.

I think I was around five years old when I received my first caning and not much older when I was given the "slipper" (on my bare bottom). Our headmaster, who would often teach the French class was a disciplinarian; a brutal man, I felt at the time, but looking back, and considering the antics I was guilty of, I think he was evenhanded. Punishments were issued without hesitation— the cane was better than the "slipper" (unless he found the comic, I stuffed down my shorts and/or he made you hold your hand knuckle side up which hurt way more than fleshy side up). To make matters worse, he made a point of performing the act in front of the rest of the class who, willingly, were teasing me and cheering him on— their main motive of course, was to try to make me cry on the way back to my desk. Most times I managed to put on a brave face and stoic expression which gave me a bit of a tough guy image and helped keep the bullies at bay.

This extrovert persona stayed with me into married life to the extent that I often enjoyed taking the lead role in family discussions but then the stroke came along, and it all changed. It was made worse because we raised our children to speak up and be enthusiastic conversation contributors. Despite the desire to actively partake in group conversations, nowadays, I cannot get a word in edgeways! It gets really frustrating hence the need to voice this irritation with the pen.

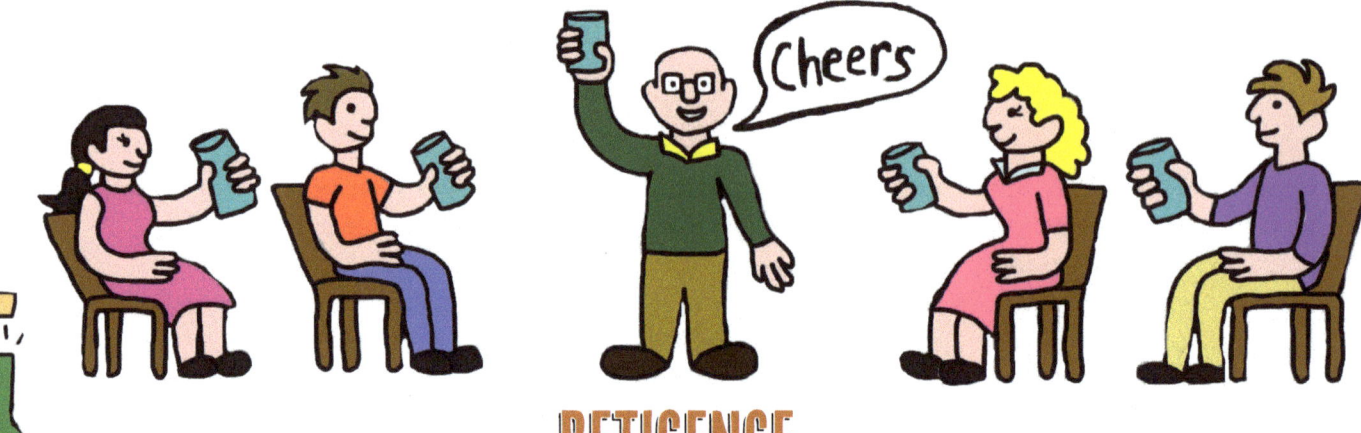

RETICENCE

When the family got together, we would sit and talk,
I used to take center stage, and nobody would balk,

Nowadays it's not so easy when the kids all come around,
I'm timid in the corner, inept to make a sound,

My speed of thought is much slower now and not at all astute,
When I finally have something to add, it's too late to contribute,

"We've moved on now Dad!" they say, when I finally get to comment,
Best I shut up and listen, regretfully I lament,

But then it's not so bad to be quiet as a church mouse,
Better than the previous me, that PATRIARCHAL LOUD-MOUTH!

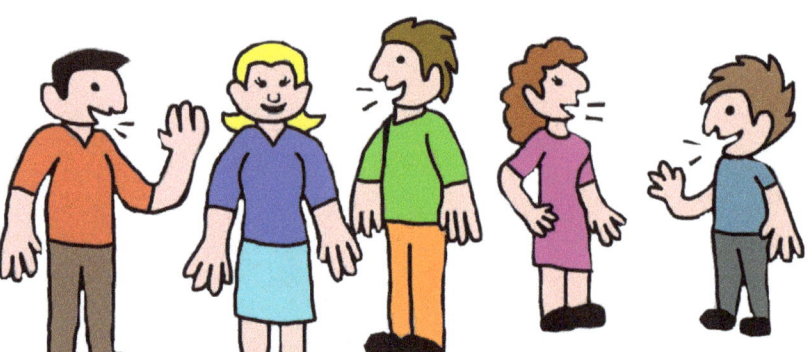

12. MY MATE KEITH

As a Brit, the single biggest thing I miss, from the "old country", is my local pub—the place that me and my mates would meet over a pint (of beer), talk about the good old days and complain about our employer, our "other halves" (spouses) or our football team's performance the week before—pathetic really. Still, it was a place to go and invariably a good night out that didn't cost the earth.

How fortunate was I that the coach of my son's local soccer team, Keith Robinson, was from Scunthorpe in the northeast of England (an ex-professional player himself) and he was in need of an assistant coach to join him on the sidelines.

It was a toss-up each week as to which one of us would get sent off by the (overly sensitive) Referee—America has not yet fully appreciated that calling out and ridiculing the referee, is very much part of the game of football—either by the coach or by the supporters in the stands. I am not sure that we set a particularly good example to our boys on the field—but they seem to have survived the ordeal without too many lasting psychological issues (I think).

Keith and I would meet for a pub evening every other Tuesday at a mutually convenient Irish pub (equi-distant between us) invariably to chat about our love of soccer and what was happening in the English Premier League (EPL). Keith followed Manchester United, and I stayed faithful to my London based, Tottenham Hotspur team and there was always some bit of gossip with one of them that dominated the conversation. Besides, when I told my cardiologist one time when I was going off to visit family in England and looking forward to a pint of (real) beer he answered along the lines, "Good for you Simon, of course, beer is an excellent diuretic and certainly won't do you any harm." As far as I was concerned, that that was clear medical advice telling me I should drink more beer. Accordingly, following the stroke and once I could get myself there and back, I saw no good reason to curtail the activity! I am also pleased to report that over the years, I have managed to educate the bar staff to only serve my beer in an "unfrosted" glass (no longer do I need to wear a glove on my right hand!).

At the time of writing, we are right in the middle of the second wave of this COVID-19 Pandemic disaster, I say "disaster" because the pub has been closed for an eternity which means I don't get to meet up with my old mate, Keith, which is almost the end of the world! I guess "absence makes the beer taste nicer" (or something like that?). Considering our pub is an Irish one, I felt it was a good time for another Limerick…

Tragically, just prior to publication, Keith lost his battle with the cancer he had been valiantly fighting the past couple of years and was taken away from his family and friends; he was a terrific bloke, and will be missed terribly—and particularly down at the pub we used to frequent!

He did read this chapter and gave me his permission to use it in the book, I am only sorry he didn't get to see and receive the final (published) version. I chose not to tamper with the ending of the poem, since metaphorically, as I continue going to the pub, in his absence, I will forever "hoist one" on his behalf and remember the many fun times we had together.

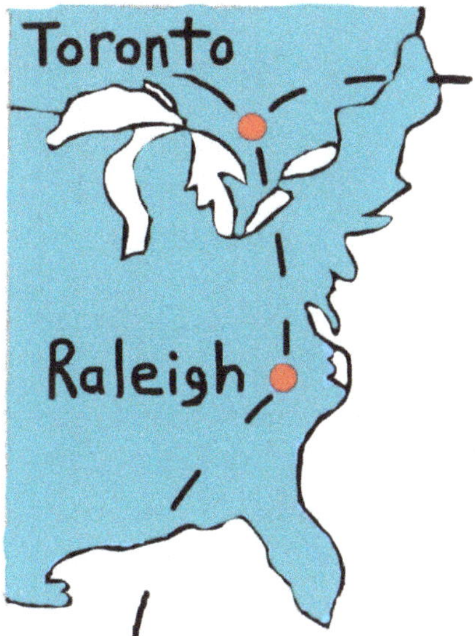

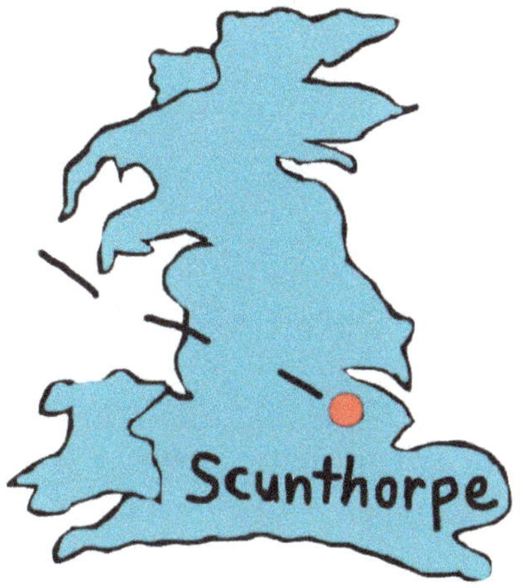

MY MATE KEITH

Keith, as a younger man, moved to Canada,
From his home in England, the distance was very far,

He got very lonely Until he met Joannie,
And despite being home-a-lot,
I still get to see him at the bar!

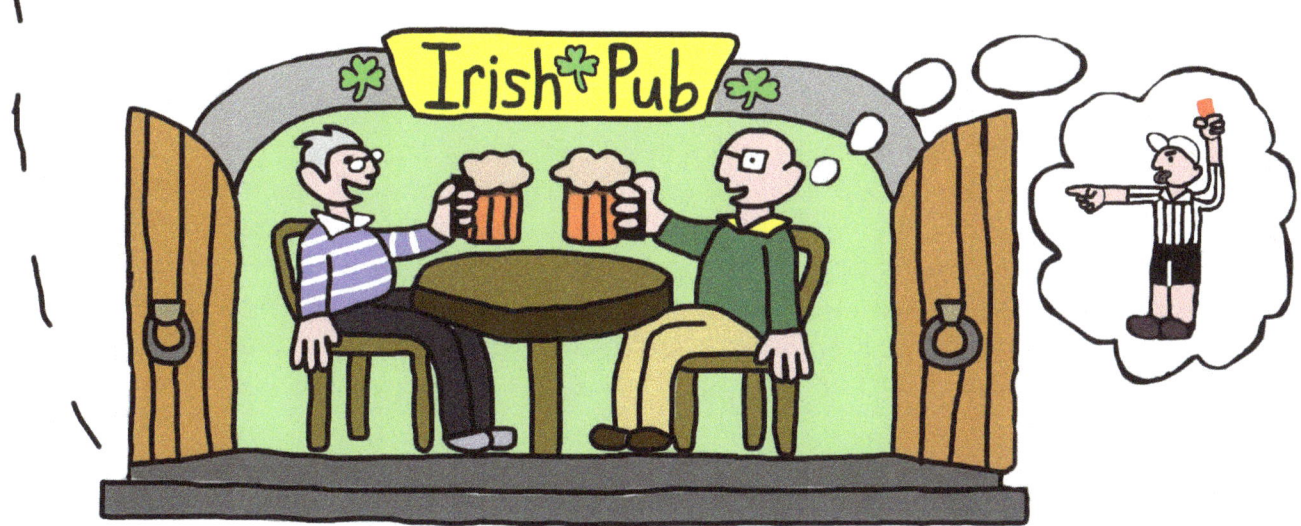

Reflections, Ramblings & Rantings of a Rancorous Stroke Survivor

13. JUST A GLIMPSE

The very same week that my mate, Keith, passed away, we lost another special friend, Ms. Joelle Marie Sarada Rogers. She was just 52 years old at the time.

Like me, Joelle was a member of TAP, but unlike me, Joelle suffered a left hemisphere hemorrhagic stroke which not only affected her mobility (hemiplegia to her right-side limbs), but she was impacted with aphasia and her ability to communicate verbally was extremely (and visibly) limited. On top of that, she had the added hardship of being diagnosed with cancer shortly after I met her. Despite the severity and extent of her difficulties, she never complained, smiled her way through the pain and on behalf of TAP, volunteered to lead their "chair yoga" class and then the meditation class for the benefit of other stroke survivors on Saturday afternoons.

Regrettably, I only knew her a short while, but I was consistently amazed and inspired by the efforts (and improvements) she made to her speech over this five to six year period—sadly, despite her fight and determination, the cancer took her away from us all.

I will never forget the many group therapy meetings we had and despite her diminutive stature, her presence was massive. Literally the moment she limped through that door with the ear to ear grin welded to her face singing, "sorry I'm late", was the same instant that a calm fell upon the group—comforted in the knowledge that all was well and now we really can begin the meeting. Over those first two to three years, I witnessed her extraordinary progress, particularly with her speech fluency. It was quite remarkable and although I am sure that pre stroke she would have spoken faster, gone were the stammers and lengthy pauses as she struggled to search for the right word. Over the next couple of years, her delivery became controlled, deliberate and flawless—a true role model to us all. I used to attend her meditation class on Saturday afternoons and found the exercise soothing and rejuvenating largely due to Joelle's thoughtfulness and eloquence. Maura, TAP's founder/director wanted each of us that attended her class to provide some kind of "one-line" tribute/reference she could use to help promote the benefits of the class and bolster the attendance. In response, I offered, "The aphasia that once made her voice disappear has now become the voice I long to hear." A more true and sincere statement, I could not conjure.

During the winter of 2020, I was invited to provide a talk about my poststroke journey to graduating SLP students at Appalachian State University and Joelle, having previously worked as a marriage guidance counselor in the town of Boone, asked to hitch a ride to visit with some friends there.

Along the way, she asked me how I was feeling and whether I was confident with my presentation. I made mention that I was a little nervous about a joke I had tailored to tell, since I had never used it before —especially on a new and young audience. Without hesitation, Joelle said, "Try your joke on me, since I will be impartial and give you an honest answer." Imagine my disappointment when I gave her my very best pitch only to find that after delivering the punch line, she barely raised the hint of a smile, after a few seconds pondering and head-scratching, she turned to me with a deadpan face and said, "it was good, you should keep it in." sensing my continued doubt she added, "no, seriously Simon, I think they will like it, keep it in." again with little to no emotion or enthusiasm.

Rather than me simply dropping her off at her friend's house, Joelle said she wanted to be in the audience to witness my presentation, which was "fine by me," I responded.

After arriving at the auditorium, I proceeded to set up and get familiar with the visual and audio facilities while Joelle took her seat, front row, left of center. Once the students took their seats and were settled and the professor introduced me, I was off doing my thing!

Most of my talk was a bit of a blur but just over halfway through I remember quite clearly that moment when, at the appointed time, I introduced my funny story with, "which reminds me … did you hear about the grizzly bear with aphasia that walks into a bar?" Within a split second of me giving the punch line, I was greeted with a unanimous wave of spontaneous laughter that filled the room. But laughing the loudest by far was this little lady sitting in the front row just left of center. When our eyes met, Joelle winked at me with that "I told you so" expression on her face.

I knew Joelle for barely ten percent of her life and less than ten percent of mine, it was the shortest of spells—barely a glimpse into the life of someone that was the true definition of a free spirit, multi-layered, generous to a fault, fascinating and very special that should have taken a lifetime to unravel … I will never forget her and the way she inspired me (and others around her). I certainly will never forget that brief time we shared together on our day trip to Boone, North Carolina on a snowy day in February 2020.

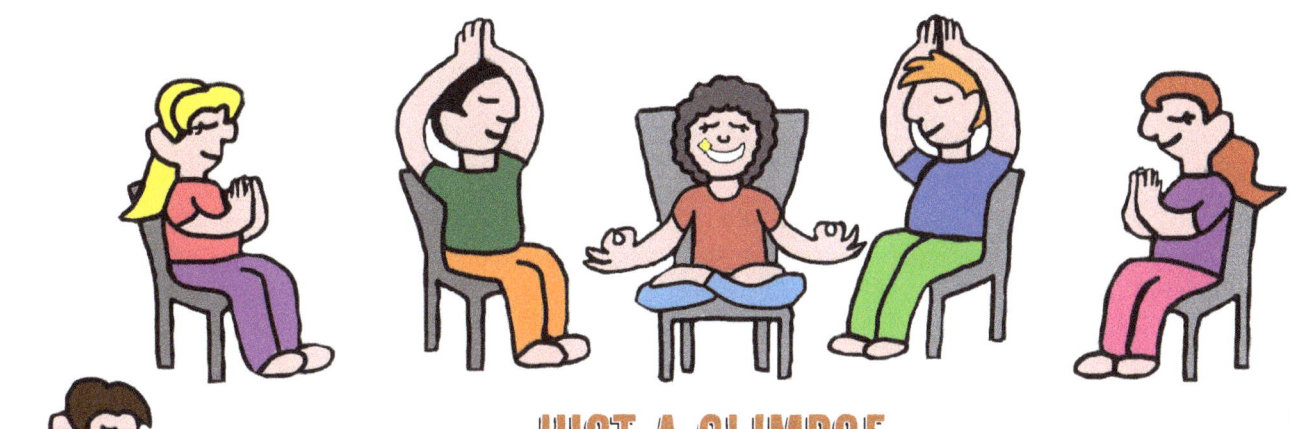

JUST A GLIMPSE

Just a glimpse of your smile as it danced around the room,
The scratch to your scalp as you contemplated,
That glint in your eye as you worked it all out,
Just glimpses, maybe, often understated.

Just a glimpse of the crease in your cheeks as you laughed 'til you burst,
That angled brow when you doubted the reason.
The kiss from your lips as you quenched your thirst,
Just glimpses, maybe, with utmost expletion.

For just a glimpse we were witnesses to you,
Shortest while but memory trove, lifetime long,
Despite all your strife's, by letting us view,
Glimpses collected, have made us so strong.

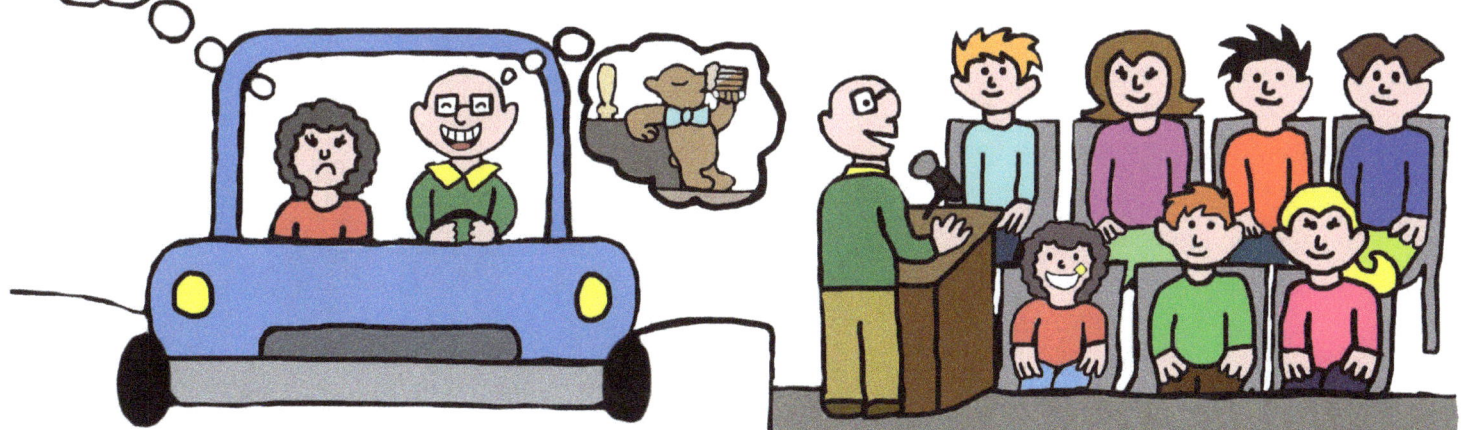

14. ROTTEN ENDINGS

It's funny how everything seemed so simple just a few years ago. I feel that sometime during the year 2013, someone (or something) pulled a lever and made everything way too complicated which happened to coincide with my medical event, which itself, was also like someone (or something) pulling a lever in my head that made me become particularly stupid!

I always loved going to the movies or even staying at home and watching a good, exciting story unfold on the box. The fact that my family and friends do not seem to experience the same difficulties I struggle with suggests that the answer to this irritation is more with the latter argument (me) rather than the former statement (the conspirators), sadly. But heck, as the grumpy cantankerous old geezer I have become (and it is my book afterall), I am still entitled to have a dig if I choose—and this next subject along with the poem that immediately follows associated with watching movies, are right at the top of my "things that piss me off, list"!

I have always been a "happy-ending" sort of guy. I know in my heart that me and my new self are going to be just fine and dandy when I get to and wherever it is I am going. I really don't care to see those endings where the villain gets away with it or the principal man and woman don't get to walk off into the sunset holding hands; I have no time for those movies where the director is looking for some kind of artistic creativity resulting in an unpredictable and disappointing conclusion or how they want to set us up for a sequel movie to follow.

Stroke survivors refuse to believe they are victims and spend their recovery time looking forward to seeing their poststroke journeys conclude having contributed to society and the wellbeing of others along the way—another happy ending, of course!

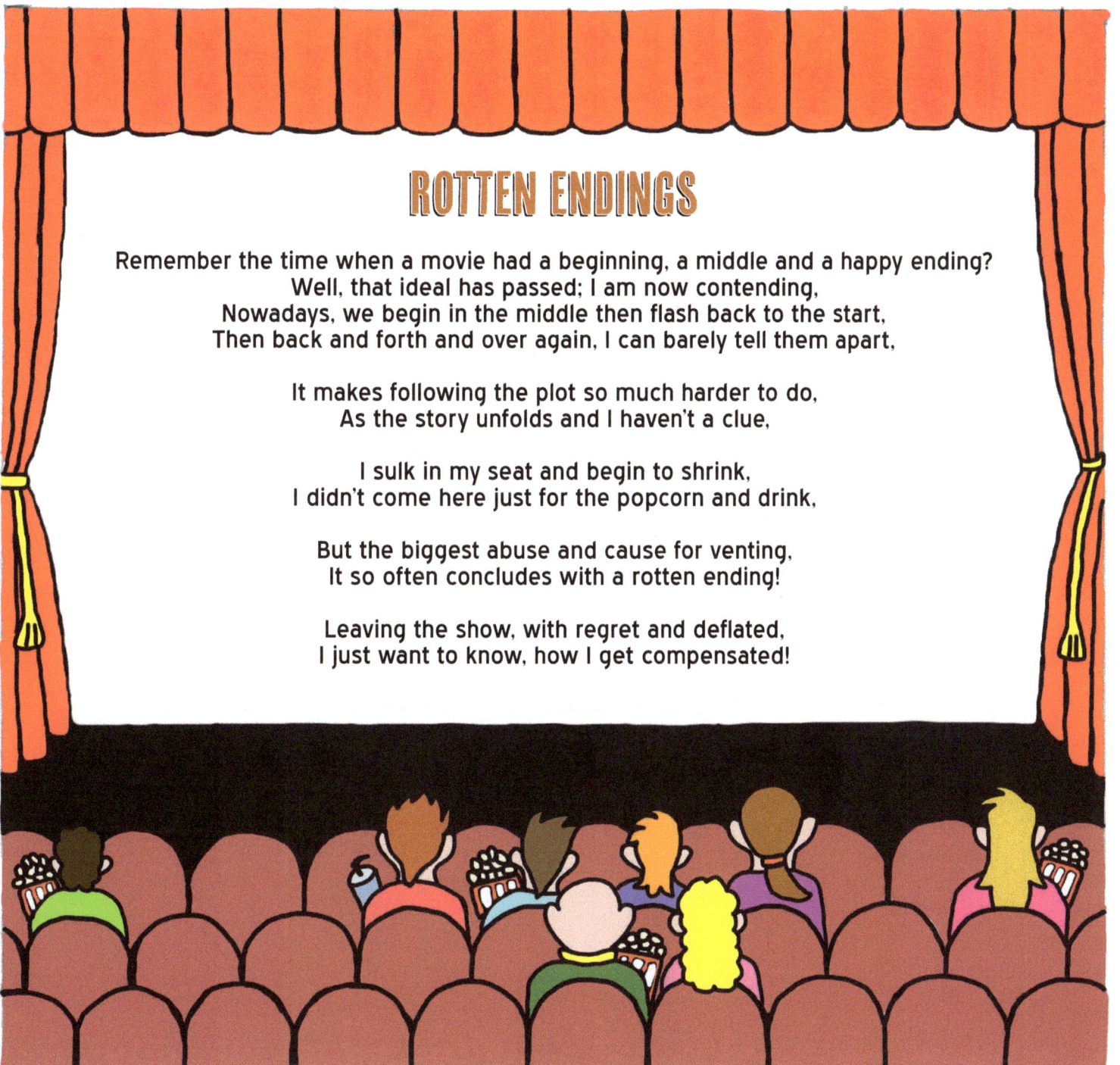

ROTTEN ENDINGS

Remember the time when a movie had a beginning, a middle and a happy ending?
Well, that ideal has passed; I am now contending,
Nowadays, we begin in the middle then flash back to the start,
Then back and forth and over again, I can barely tell them apart,

It makes following the plot so much harder to do,
As the story unfolds and I haven't a clue,

I sulk in my seat and begin to shrink,
I didn't come here just for the popcorn and drink,

But the biggest abuse and cause for venting,
It so often concludes with a rotten ending!

Leaving the show, with regret and deflated,
I just want to know, how I get compensated!

15. MURDER MYSTERY MAYHEM

Following on from the previous chapter, my complaint at watching movies these days is not just limited to the theater but extends to the comfort of my own home!

Sarah and I love to watch a good "who done it" type murder mystery on the box. But again, I fear today's screenwriters like to make it really hard for the "cognitively challenged" audience. So many times, I have given up by episode three of a six episode series. Since this appears to be the new norm, it is probably best that I get busy writing one myself!

Since the stroke, Sarah is convinced I have become more "OCD" in my manner. Just the way I have to be methodical in all the things I do and how I do them, and anything that requires a little initiative on my part is frequently doomed to fail.

Should she place a bottle of milk in front of my breakfast yoghurt in the fridge then I will likely go without. Far be it for me to actually move things around to look behind! If it was visible yesterday and I cannot see it today, then we must have run out. With that level of competence, how on earth am I supposed to follow something where the crime story was based around some kind of complex conspiracy driven plot, and when the villain is not the one wearing the black and white striped shirt with a balaclava over his head carrying the bag on his shoulder marked "LOOT". Equally stereotypical these days, if the bad guy is not the one speaking in a clipped English accent, then how on earth am I supposed to spot them?

As implied earlier, it is made harder when we watch one of those "streaming" (made for TV) series. I now have to remember what happened three or four episodes earlier, 2 weeks ago! Impossible.

If you can relate to this dilemma, imagine how it must be for my wife, doing her best to enjoy and follow the story herself only to get constantly interrupted by the bloke next to her twittering on, "remind me the film we saw that actor in recently?" and, "why did she leave him?" Occasionally Sarah will eventually lose her cool and put me in my place, rolling her eyes as she responds gruffly, "probably for the same reason I'm going to be leaving you, if you don't shut up!"

MURDER MYSTERY MAYHEM

Watching a "who done it movie" can be quite a chore,
It's very hard to follow and can make my brain feel sore,

Usually my wife is sitting there, right next to me,
Before I can ask, "who did what to whom?" she's gone to make the tea.

As she returns, she asks, "what happened while I was away?"
"Sorry dear," I answer, "my mind had gone astray."

She should know it's preferable, not to leave at such a vital time,
When I'm totally incapable, to follow this bloomin' crime!

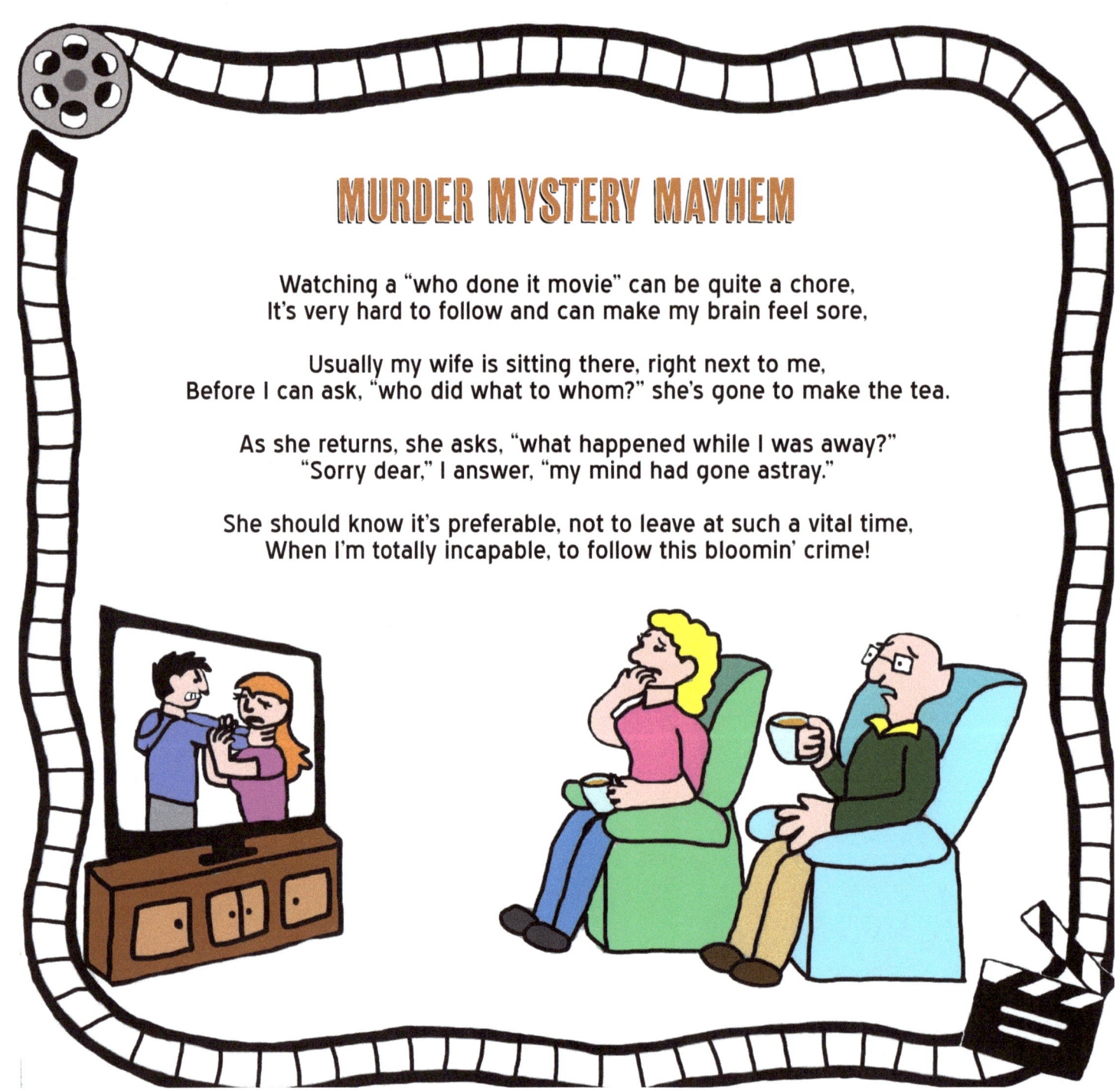

16. LIFE'S QUARTERLY HIGHLIGHTS

My dear old dad used to think in terms of life quarters on the basis that by today's standards our lives are made up of four (metric) quarters; 0-25 being the first when we are born and when we are totally green about everything and concluding with the fourth quarter (75-100) when we are older and wiser, a little "filter less" and carefree and the period when we are more likely to pass on and meet our maker (for those who have been good, that is).

I remember Dad in his eighties still playing quite a good round of golf but on the rare occasion he hit a bad shot into the trees he would turn to his playing partners and with a smirk on his face, would quip, "What do you expect? I am in my fourth quarter you know!" Likewise, he would use the same expression if he bumped the curb when parking or dribbling some soup onto his tie, passing wind in earshot of others and so the list went on.

I have found myself using the same formula consistently since my stroke—which of course is now well into my third quarter (although, since the stroke, it feels I have been propelled into the fourth)—on the basis that any of the quarters are capable of having those occasional ups and downs, moments—when it is "up" then the phrase can still be used it just morphs into, "not bad for someone in his third quarter, don't you think?" Although, these days I prefer to remember the highlights rather than the downsides of each quarter, hence the more positive message within the following poem, I hope you agree …

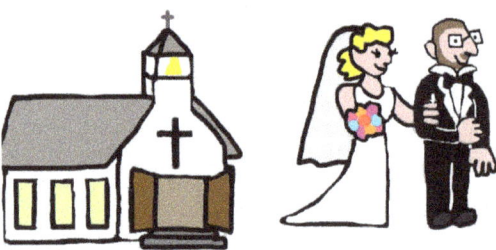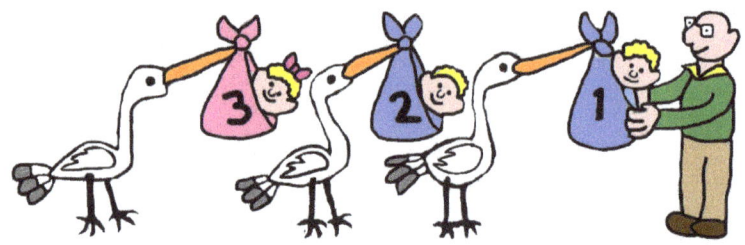

LIFE'S QUARTERLY HIGHLIGHTS

My first quarter was fun, As I learned about life,
And highlighted by finding the perfect wife.

Second quarter focused on growing the family,
Three kids soon came, all huge highlights, understandably,

The third quarter was time to seek a new fate,
The highlight came with a job in the States.
Despite the adventure, "living the dream" became fantasy,
When the period was marred by a health catastrophe.

The stroke I suffered can never be undone,
Quite soon, I discovered, my fourth quarter had begun!

But life remains bright, as you will all gather,
Such is the highlight of becoming a grandfather.

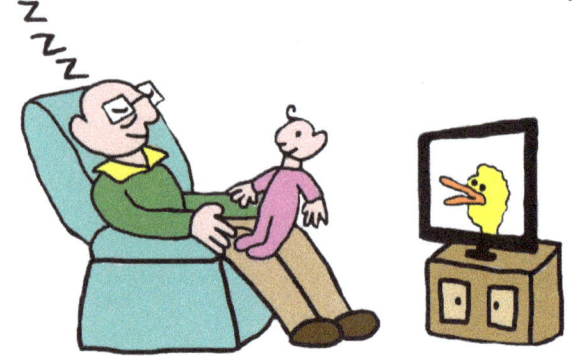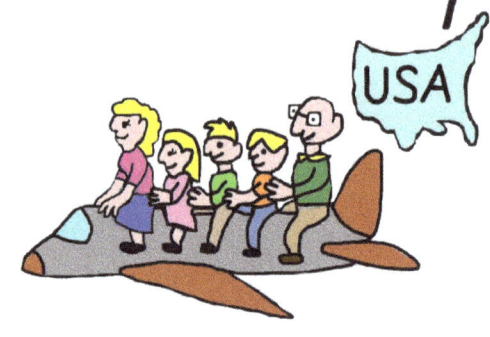

BAD RHYMES, NO REASON

17. NEURO-FATIGUE

During my stay in rehab hospital, it seemed like I was more asleep than awake. On more than one occasion I would awake to find a note left on my pillow by a visiting friend that read, "just dropped by, didn't want to wake you, see you next time, keep fighting, much love, etc., etc..."

When I was eventually sent home, and particularly that first year, I got really tired to the point that Sarah only had to put the TV on and within moments, I was, head back, mouth open, catching ZZ's. As time progressed then the timing and extent of my rest depended on how much I was trying to do, I found. I could not go more than two to three hours at a time before feeling the need to close my eyes somewhere. Early on, my average day involved a couple of physical therapy sessions only, but as I became cognitively stronger and felt the need to add in some office time then it seemed my lethargy worsened. Apparently, this symptom is quite common following the type of brain injury I received, quite normal and in medical terms, is known as "Neuro-fatigue".

The good news is that it does improve; the bad news is that as it improves, the more (you feel) you need to do, which just makes you as mentally weary as before! (Seems you cannot win). But there is no doubt I am doing much more these days and less dependent on napping; at least, compared with years one to three post. I find I can do my twenty-minute walk in the morning followed by a mid-morning session in the office of one to two hours and another after lunch. I still take advantage for an occasional afternoon break, but it is nowhere near as long nor as regimental as it used to be.

This need to close one's eyes is not a bad thing, as my neurologist told me early on, "it is just the brain saying, 'I need to shut down and recuperate for a bit', so don't deny the process," she said.

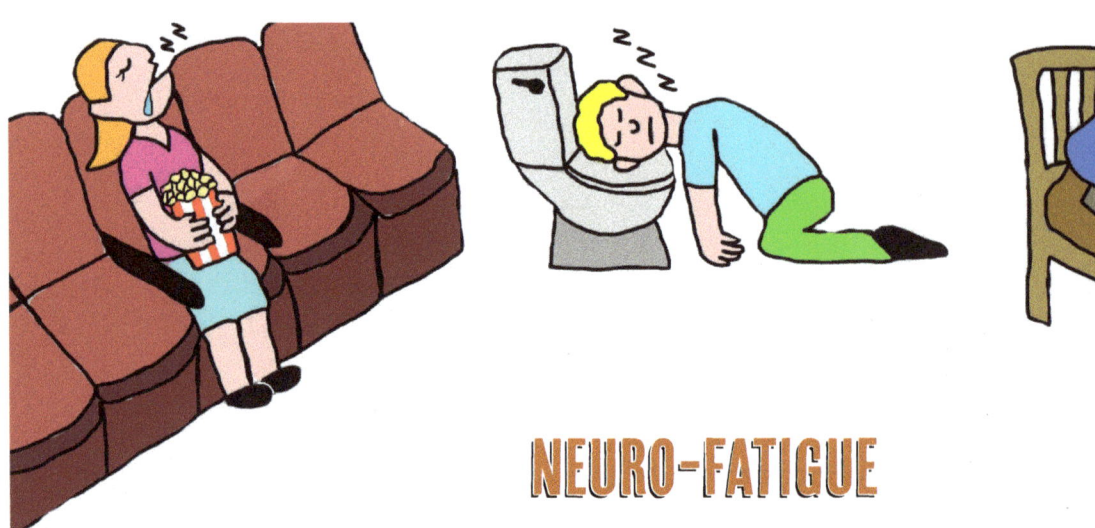

NEURO-FATIGUE

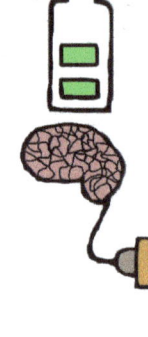

It is okay to nap when you tire,
A daily snooze helps your brain re-wire,
Work with no relief can be quite a chore,
It's tough to achieve, what you did before,

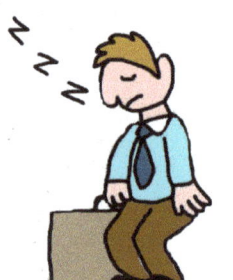

When the day stinks and goes demanding,
Take forty winks or even doze while standing,
When you are not mentally strong with no access to a mattress,
Putting off sleep too long, could be disastrous,

Nobody could possibly blame you,
They have no idea what your brain has been through,
There's no conspiracy; no reason for intrigue,
The condition is real and called "Neuro fatigue!"

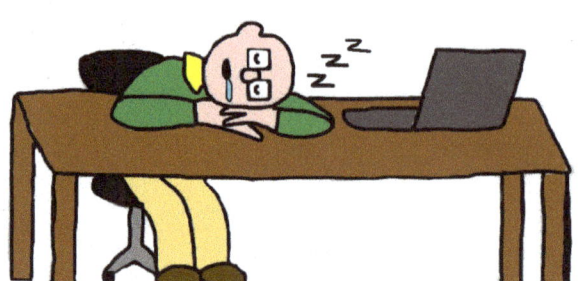
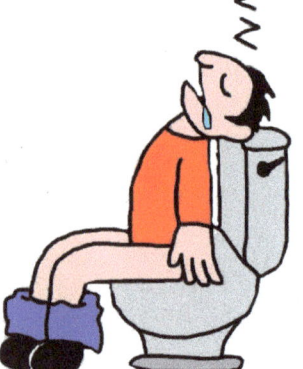

BAD RHYMES, NO REASON

18. INSPIRATION

On those occasions I get the opportunity to present my journey story, the question I am most asked is, "what factor(s) have been the biggest and most positive influence on [my] recovery journey to date?" For me, there has only ever been one answer: "Other stroke survivors!". In the Triangle area of North Carolina where I live, I have been most fortunate to join and/or become part of a number of stroke/brain injury support groups—mostly organized and chaired by an exceptionally dedicated and talented (therapist type) Professional but the rest made up of brain injury survivors, just like me. As I have said before, many have their own set of complications they must battle. But without exception, every meeting I attend I usually come away having learned something new and without fail, inspired by the stories shared by the attendees. I can honestly say, these meetings are very much part of the undetermined journey I have been following and as mentioned in chapter 3. "The Journey" – the people I refer to as being "fun to be around".

It is not unusual to find that a growing distance appears between the friends we had before our injury, but that fact is only natural and does not stop us from making new friends. Our respective struggles give us something in common and serve as a platform and guide to help us deal with the future.

Certainly, we are often moved and motivated by many of the medical professionals we have all had the good fortune to meet but I cannot pay tribute enough to the many new (stroke survivor) friends I have made who themselves experience, daily, many of the complaints (and more) I have had to endure.

So, to all of you stroke survivors out there, and particularly my colleagues at the "Back to Work Group" of the TAP organization I support, thank you! This next poem is for you!

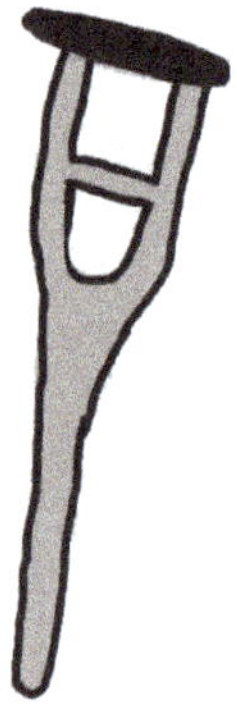

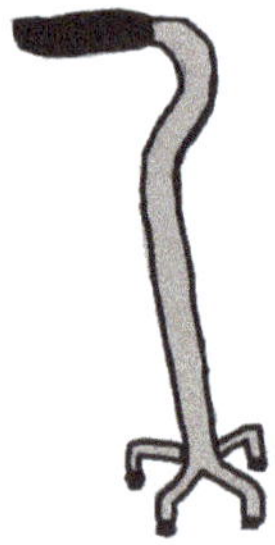

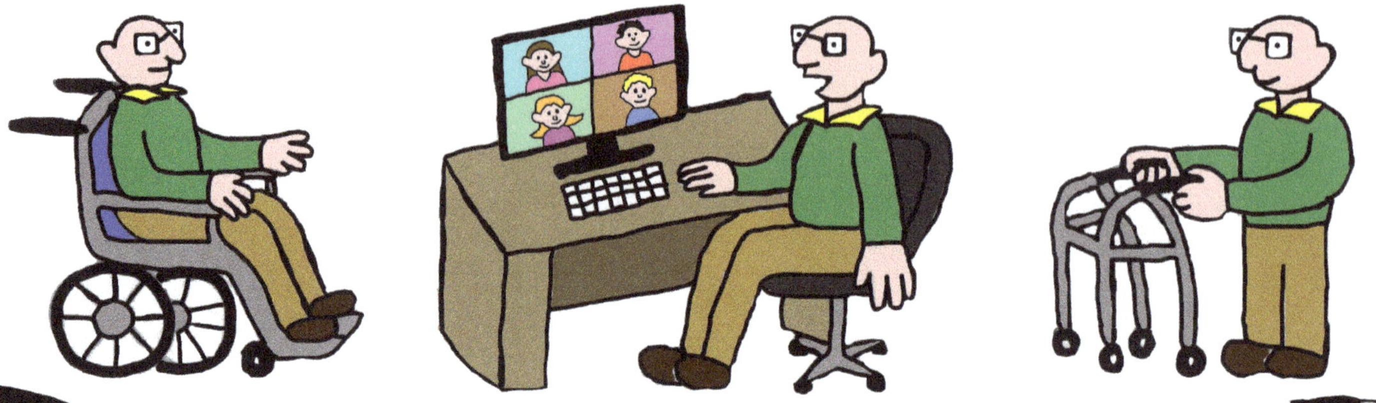

INSPIRATION

I emphasized when I had my stroke, we would be on our own,
Pleasantly surprised to have misspoken, for we were not alone,

With my concerns, others there are many,
Along with local support groups, resources are aplenty,

My early thoughts of doom and gloom were prematurely mistaken,
For these lovely people and groups, have become my inspiration,

So, thank you fellow survivors, you have helped me on my way,
Continue being fighters, all will be okay.

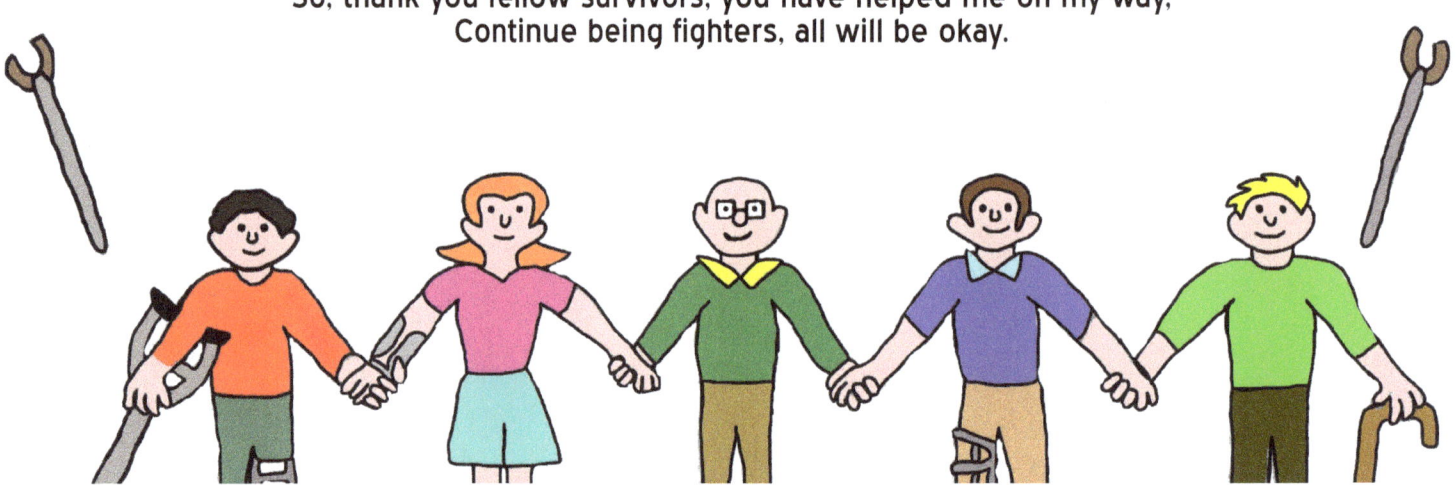

19. OH TO SING

One of the many good things to come out of this rotten event is that it gave me the opportunity to rediscover my relationship with God. My eldest son, Josh, got married the week after I was admitted to hospital and I missed the service but was kindly wheeled (horizontal) to the following reception—all thanks to the fabulous nurses that were taking care of me at the time, and prepared to break a rule (or three)!

It so happens that the wedding was conducted at a local Methodist church, whose denomination is not that far removed from the Church of England I was raised and confirmed within as a boy and certainly, a lot closer than the Baptist teachings that tend to dominate the churches of North Carolina and the southern states that I never managed to embrace. Anyway, I was a little nervous but plucked up the courage to go along one Sunday morning and was delighted to receive a very kind welcome not only from the Pastor but by many within the congregation.

As it turns out, I felt it important that I reestablish my connection with the almighty one, for some reason (and we know He moves in mysterious ways), He felt it fitting to spare me that day in 2013 and give me another chance to make amends for the many screw ups I made first go around.

I must confess, however, the biggest highlight of going to church is the opportunity to sing in unison with others. Sadly, as it turned out, this was much harder than I remembered. First, with just one functional hand, it seemed to take an eternity to thumb my way to the correct page in the hymn book, and by the time I got there, I would eventually join the music sometime between the third and fourth verses! Secondly, the reasonable singing voice (I thought I had), had since been hijacked by some kind of out-of-tune-droning imposter! Thank goodness on the first couple of occasions I detected the anomaly before I got too close to others in the pews thus allowing me the opportunity to distance myself and perfect my volume control!

As time moved on, I felt bad that I was not "doing my bit" when it came to volunteering to assist with some of the chores the church needed doing—particularly those that are involved in some kind of physical effort, raking leaves and tidying up the place, etc. So, I applied (and was accepted) for the role of one of the Liturgists required to provide the Old Testament reading during each service. With a little time to prepare in advance and print out the words with large font on a single sheet of paper, I was more than capable of reading the scripture in a clear and strong voice. I was instructed that the reading takes place immediately following the first hymn and advised to start making my way to the chancel by the end of the second verse so that I was prepared and ready to go immediately following. Unfortunately, on one such occasion I was so absorbed by the hymn that I forgot my duty and didn't set off until after the third verse; the hymn had ended when I was barely halfway up the side ramp travelling at the "speed of Simon". Talk about "suspense"! Once I got to the lectern, I was conscious of all the eyes looking in my direction, I still had to remove my everyday (prism) glasses and replace with my readers. You could cut the air with a knife! "Good morning!" I said, panting, "Today's reading is …" As I left the church somewhat disappointed with myself, the pastor kindly said, "not to worry Simon, your accent won them over by the end of the reading, you did alright". Following that experience, the pastor invited me to sit next to him before the service begins, now I get to enjoy the hymn in its entirety and reach the lectern more punctually. Phew, problem solved!

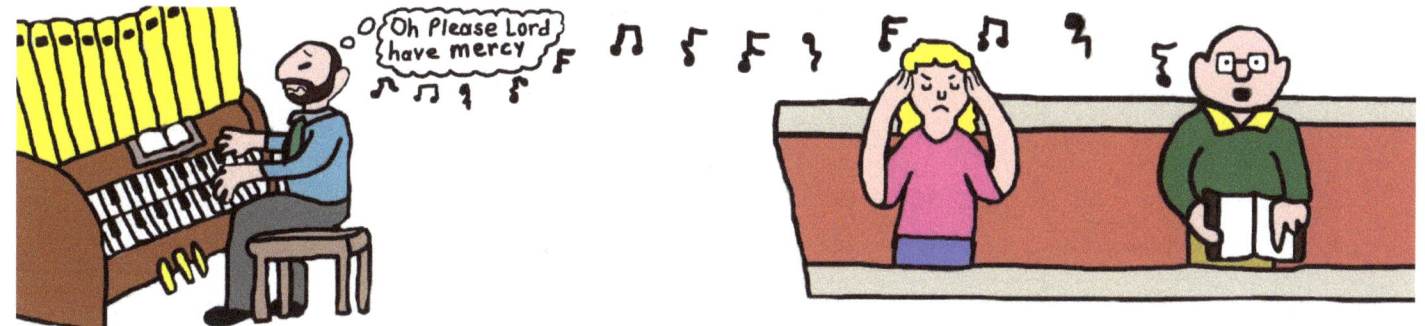

OH TO SING

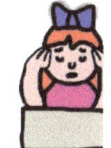

I was once a good singer, I could certainly hold a note,
Since a medical mishap, there's been something in my throat,
On Sundays I like to go to church, to listen, sing and pray,
With making such an awful din, I now sit far away,

It's very sad considering, you are there to rejoice,
With everyone else, we should sing, with no care, at top of voice!

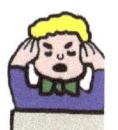

But I'm not too concerned, I don't go totally without,
Through practice, I have learned, mouthing words and "nought" coming out!

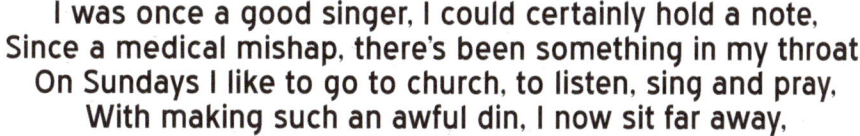
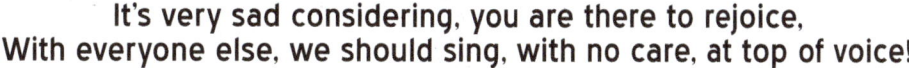

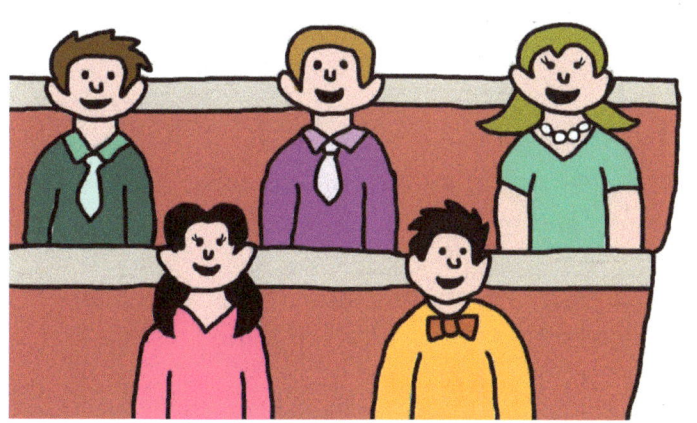
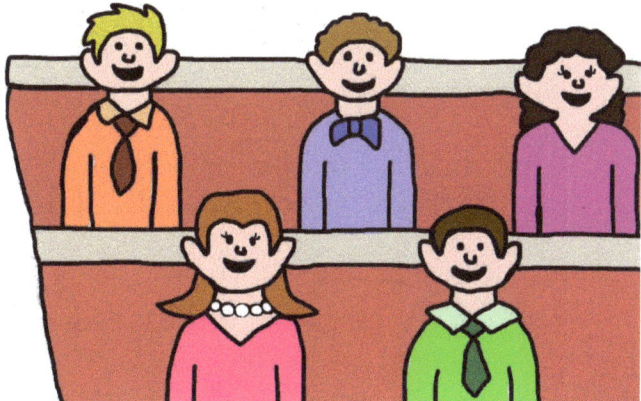

Reflections, Ramblings & Rantings of a Rancorous Stroke Survivor

20. CANTATA

Continuing the music theme a little while longer (along with being a glutton for punishment)!

The church's Director of Music, Chris Dodson, a larger-than-life kind of guy with a big beard and toothy grin (imagine the perfect 'Pantomime Pirate' without the peg leg and eye-patch, well that's him), announced that he was in the process of rehearsing for the annual Christmas Cantata and the choir was looking for additional volunteers to join.

I may have had my doubts about my newly found singing capabilities, but at the same time, I can be a little reckless and not too worried about making a fool of myself; so the following week, I decided to apply and took an audition. Either Chris was really desperate to increase his numbers in the tenor section, or he took pity on me, or more likely, in this age of equal opportunity and inclusion, he didn't feel he had met his quota for tone-deaf invalids, because (miraculously) I was accepted (Go figure)!!

I used to play classical guitar and know how to read music. However, guitar musical notation appears on the treble clef stave, you might recall that notes on the lines (E,G,B,D,F) are best remembered by the phrase, "Every Good Boy Deserves Fudge", I never had to learn the bass clef which is where the tenor's notes reside and where the same notes on the lines are evoked by the phrase, "Good Boys Do Fine Always" (G, B,D,F,A). Which makes me want to ask the following questions; when are boys ever good? I know I never was (as the kids I hung around were not), and who was it that created these ridiculous phrases in the first place and thought boys were good? I wonder, did they have some kind of brain injury, perhaps?

Fortunately, the three tenors already resident were very strong and did an amazing job covering for me as I tried to slink into the background and not cramp their style.

The music and participation were a lot of fun, a lovely experience and therapeutically speaking, a great benefit since it helped build confidence and just the sort of thing I needed at that time of my journey.

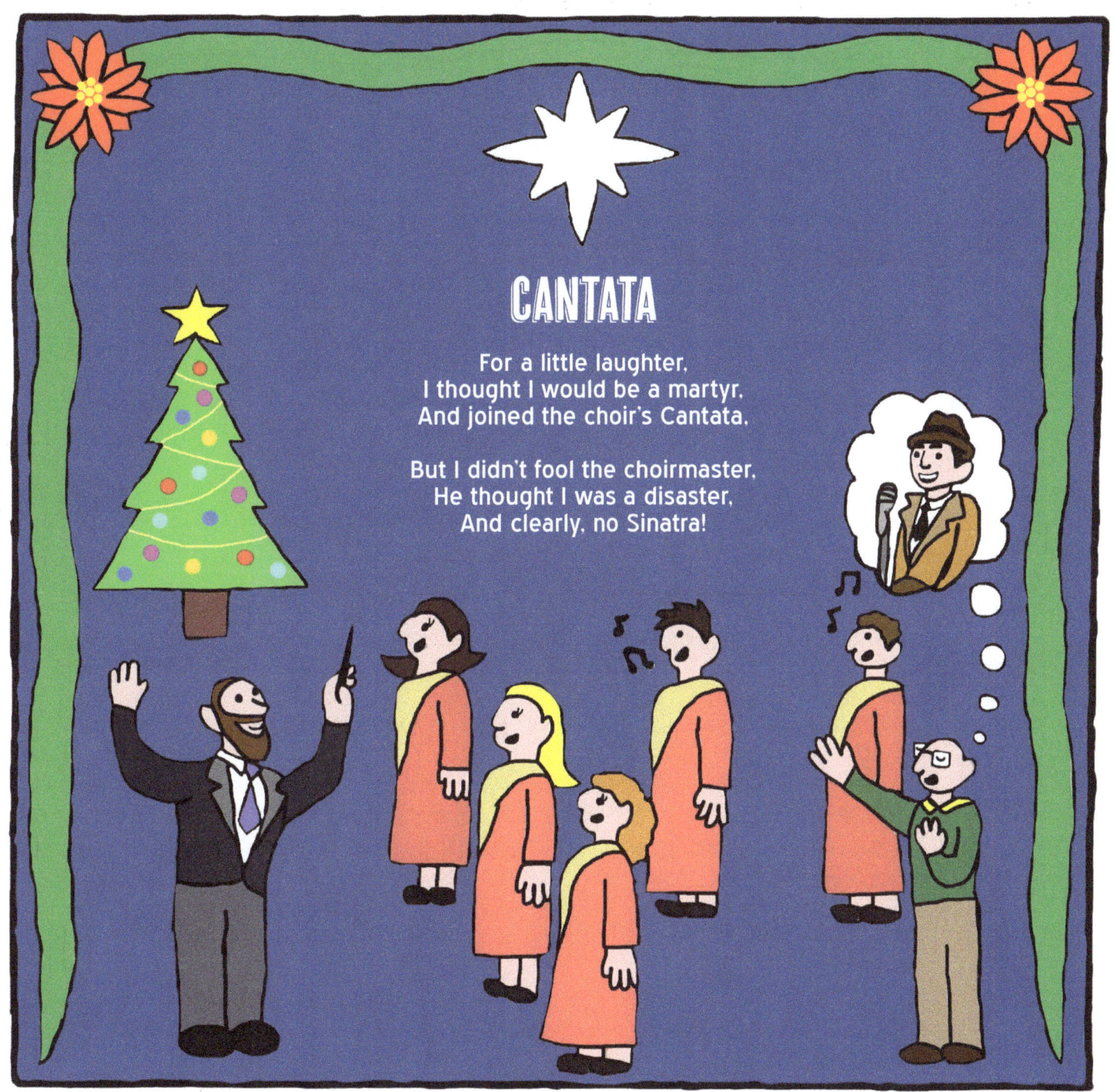

21. THAT OTHER 4-LETTER F-WORD

2016 was an interesting year—having lost my business the year before and filed for bankruptcy, I was now officially unemployed (the first time in my adult life). I successfully managed to be approved for Social Security Disability Allowance, courtesy of "Uncle Sam". This certainly helped but could not possibly sustain us in the house that we had come to love over the previous twenty years. Sarah was already working crazy hours to help make ends meet, but we had to take the plunge and down-size. We needed to sell up and move to a smaller, easier to manage and more affordable abode and the sooner, the better!

That same year we had two major political events. In June, the UK was having a referendum to determine whether or not to leave the European Union which was followed by the American general election in November to decide our next president.

In both cases, expectations as purported by the mainstream media were hopelessly underestimated. First, it was decided by a referendum majority 52:48% that the United Kingdom should leave the European Union and a couple of months later, Donald J. Trump, more known for being a reality TV personality and (questionable) businessman than a politician, won the presidency against Hilary Clinton by 304 to 227 electoral seats. Nothing less than shock and horror filled the media waves and all kinds of excuses for both events were made to explain away the results. The resistance to these results (and ensuing arguments) continued on through the next three years on both sides of the pond.

Coincidentally, in the UK, and quite shortly after, the decision was made to adopt a new feature called "VAR" (Video Assistant Referee) for our national game of English football (soccer). This is a technology aid that had been proposed in the past and something that many of us were against on the basis that it would/could have a detrimental effect on the flow of our lovely game. Unlike many US sports, we don't have "timeouts" for commercial breaks; the match is nonstop for 45 minutes then we have a brief (fifteen-minute), half time break before concluding the game after another 45 minute (nonstop) half.

It occurred to me during this period that all three events are linked to the same root issue. In recent times, there has been a growing desire to avoid upsetting each other politically or socially to the point we now find ourselves tiptoeing our way through life for fear of stepping out of line and causing offense—the exponentially growing phenomenon of "fairness". Interestingly, the actual adoption and practical experience of VAR has not improved anything; as forecast, we now "twiddle our fingers" for a while and wait for the final decision to come along and laughingly, the fans still think it is the wrong decision and it is still so unfair! (Boohoo).

My earliest memories of expressing my feelings of being hard done by, was met with a quick and sharp kind of scolding which usually concluded with one of my parents rebuking, "life is not FAIR, so get over it!". I remember my first (and only) tennis coach telling me that "the true dignity of a sportsman is best measured by the behavior they exhibit after losing a tough match," he then went on emphasizing, "regardless of how well you (or they) played, you shake their hands at the end and say, 'good game, well played!' Then proceed to the changing room with your head held high—nothing more, nothing less!" Is this level of sportsmanship really an ideal that can no longer be attained? It has been my experience, that as with many ardent sports team fans that are so partisan, they can be blinded by reality; it has often been the case, that rarely does the sports match end with a winner that didn't win under contestable circumstances. But generally speaking, we would walk away muttering negatively at the missed opportunities, wrong calls and injustices committed, but come Monday, we eventually got over it and we gathered ourselves for the next fixture the following weekend. In short, we moved on!

During our lifetimes we are frequently tested with disappointments, setbacks, and sadness; we may not get the job we applied for; we will lose a loved one to death. And, of course, some of us will suffer a serious health concern of some kind, like a stroke, for example—a medical misfortune of some kind.

According to the CDC (Centers for Disease Control), "stroke is the leading cause of serious long-term disability in America," (and I dare say, within the world). Despite this fact, of all the many stroke survivors I have had the pleasure to meet. notwithstanding the enormity of their struggles, not one have I heard complain about their predicament. They are way too busy working on their respective journeys to dwell on how unfair it all was.

Call me "old-fashioned" and "out of touch" but I am not giving up on the cause, which is why I have included the following poem in this book.

If you are offended by some of the content referenced, then maybe, I did hit the right nerve but trust me, life will go on.

THAT OTHER 4-LETTER F-WORD

"It's not FAIR!" they said,
"A Bigot in the office? With a haystack on his head?"
".. It was the Russians with whom he colluded,"
"SHE, would have been so much better instead,"
Cries to impeach, in the house, they led,
"It's just not FAIR!" they said,

"It's not FAIR!" they cried,
When the vote favored the BREXIT side,
"Xenophobes and cheats… And they lied,"
"The vote was close and should have been tied,"
"We will resist it," the Parliamentarians sighed,
".. And do our best to brush it aside,"
"It's just not FAIR!" they cried,

"It's not FAIR!" they roared,
"The ball touched a hand, before he scored,"
"A video replay will expose the fraud,"
"It's just not FAIR!" they roared.

"It's not FAIR! Was his last-ditch stake,"
"Like the news, mail-in voting is fake!"
"I won't concede, I won't let them take,"
"The Supreme Court will give me a break,"
"It's just not FAIR," he continued to stake,

Look at what the world is becoming,
Petulant children we are succumbing,

"It's not FAIR!" she choked,
When the Doctor said he had a stroke,
"It will be okay," she said in hope,
"I will roll up my sleeves and help him cope"

It's good that some still think it absurd,
To give in to this 4-letter word.

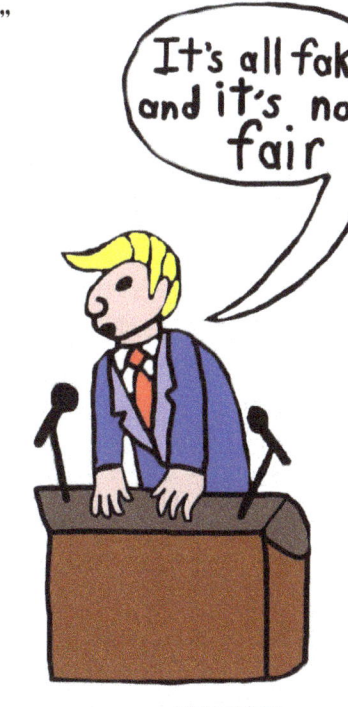

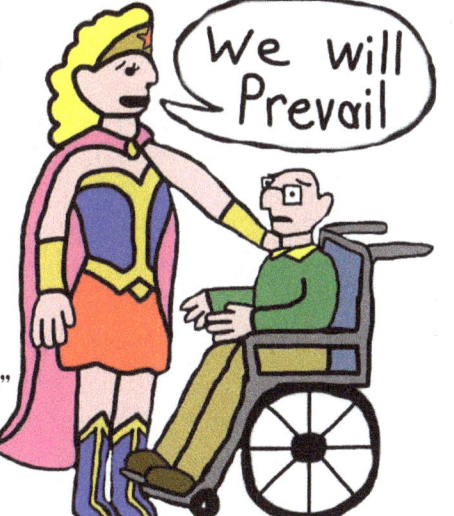

Reflections, Ramblings & Rantings of a Rancorous Stroke Survivor

22. FOG

I met with my neurologist the other day for a simple follow-up appointment. As usual, she expressed great interest and praise with those areas that were clear signs of progress and sympathized with those issues that had not improved as much as we both would have liked.

Despite the fact that I did not suffer badly with aphasia; as is often the case with me these days, I still find it quite hard to verbally express or form coherent answers to questions and particularly in group situations and where the inquirer is focused on my response and placing a little added attention to me and so, when the doctor asked about any concerns I might have relating to other symptoms I was experiencing, on this occasion, I wanted to reference the fact that I still suffer with a kind of mild form of drowsiness; yet no headaches and no real discomfort but something that has always been there from the moment I was released from hospital following the stroke event. From her bemused expression, I could see I was not getting across my point. When I got home, I tried to write it down in the hope that it might be easier and clearer to convey.

I have found that the biggest benefit to writing has been the single act of conveying a message with the content, intent and spirit required. It may take me a while to compose and type with my one good hand, but frankly, my brain needs the time to think it over anyway. Besides, the same brain certainly cannot work fast enough to express to the same clarity, verbally.

I am not sure it ever did, pre stroke either. I have always been envious of those "old-school" business professionals, like my father that could dictate a letter (start to finish) into a Dictaphone for his secretary to type up later. Winston Churchill used to dictate most of his books directly to the typist. I can undertake as many as four re-writes of just one simple paragraph, let alone a page, let alone a 1-page letter, let alone a book!

Having re-read the following poem, I am not sure it is still any clearer ... nevertheless, after receiving the poem, my neurologist took the precautionary measure of having me undergo an MRI, which, I am pleased to report showed nothing concerning, I later found out.

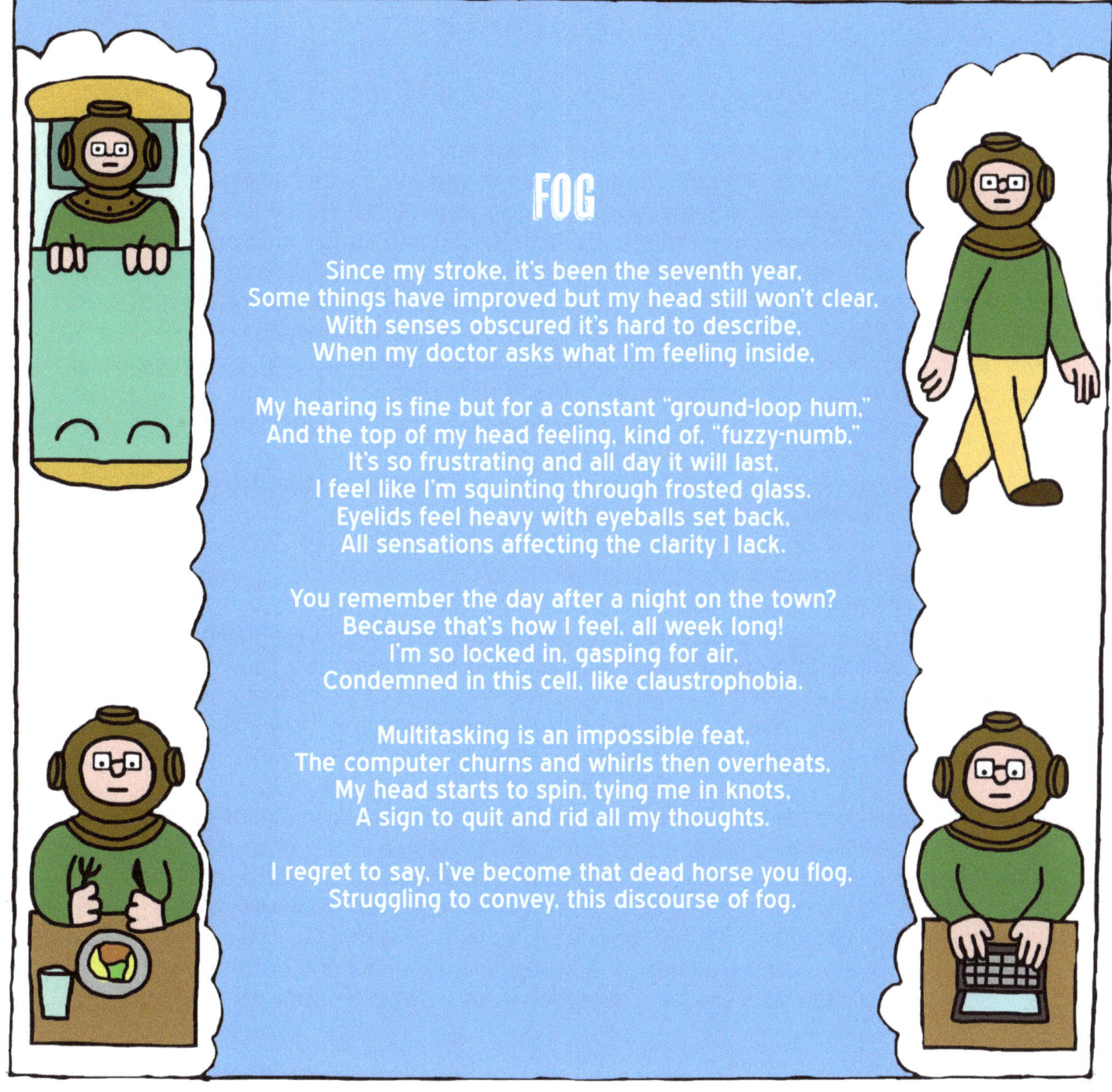

FOG

Since my stroke, it's been the seventh year,
Some things have improved but my head still won't clear,
With senses obscured it's hard to describe,
When my doctor asks what I'm feeling inside.

My hearing is fine but for a constant "ground-loop hum,"
And the top of my head feeling, kind of, "fuzzy-numb,"
It's so frustrating and all day it will last,
I feel like I'm squinting through frosted glass,
Eyelids feel heavy with eyeballs set back,
All sensations affecting the clarity I lack.

You remember the day after a night on the town?
Because that's how I feel, all week long!
I'm so locked in, gasping for air,
Condemned in this cell, like claustrophobia.

Multitasking is an impossible feat,
The computer churns and whirls then overheats,
My head starts to spin, tying me in knots,
A sign to quit and rid all my thoughts.

I regret to say, I've become that dead horse you flog,
Struggling to convey, this discourse of fog.

23. MR. DARCY

I love dogs; or should I say, I love some dogs! One of my earliest childhood memories was when I was around two or 3 years old and I tried to ram my mother's beloved Sealyham terrier, Judy, in the driveway with my new tricycle and she bit me on the knee—my mother showed absolutely no sympathy with the resulting wound and excruciating pain. As I recall, Mum took retaliatory pleasure by vigorously rubbing in the TCP Antiseptic into the open gash and watching me squirm and scream before applying the bandage uttering, "well it does serve you right, dear!" In my defense, nobody liked Judy! Even Dad when returning from a hard day's work would receive her growling welcome—he hated that dog as did my brother and sisters. As we got older the dogs got bigger and friendlier, first, a series of Labradors before moving onto Dieter—the epitome of the perfectly behaved German shepherd.

Fortunately, my wife Sarah, also liked dogs so it was only natural that they become a feature of ours and our children's lives, as our family grew.

I bought Mr. Darcy as a silver wedding anniversary gift for Sarah (some gift considering she was in charge of the morning poop scoops during his first year). My kids undertook a great deal of research helping me source him—respecting my hopes and expectations. He was a Saint Bernard with an impressive pedigree highlighted by notable past show champions in his lineage. He was just a bundle of fluff (weighing less than 10 lbs.) when I picked him up from the airport, "like an expectant father" said the cargo officer as I ran in 5 minutes after he landed at RDU.

He was not greedy nor was he a fussy eater; he was never aggressive and despite his rapid growth, fancied himself as a lap dog, practically crushing the hardiest of thighs. He was the perfect "gentle giant", he rejoiced with our best moments and sympathized through our lowest periods, and he was loved by us all. I remember him sitting patiently at the curbside when I was eventually wheeled out of rehab hospital and those first few months when I was quite incapable of anything, he did his best to keep his distance but lay close to my side in the hope of a pat on the back and some attention when I was in a position to offer it.

I had previously mentioned the important role that family and friends can play in a stroke survivor's journey to wellness; but included in that group, must be pets. My poorly mother did her bit at the end of a long-distance phone call, as did others (my over-the-pond siblings particularly). Sarah would help get me up washed and dressed each morning, help me with my therapy exercises but then she had to go to work to help pay the bills. This meant that the only remaining consistent and friendly face I had left to relate with was Darcy and faithfully he displayed the very best behavior and was never demanding and certainly not in need of anything that would be difficult for me to provide.

Sadly, he was aging really fast and at the time we had to move we suspected he was on borrowed time. The house move meant a short stay in the smallest of apartments—that was certainly way too small for the three of us (bear in mind that Mr. Darcy was around 180-200 lbs. around this time). Understandably, the rules of the apartment complex meant that all dogs had to be on a leash at all times. Despite the fact that by then I had become more confident and steadier with my walking, no way could I control him or feel secure with him on a leash should other dogs come over to say, "hello". This inevitably meant less exercise for us both.

In those short "limbo" months we saw him get much older and frailer.

We were particularly excited to find a house that not only served our needs and was affordable, but it also offered a nicely sized back yard and a space that was big enough for Darcy to go and relieve himself along with a stretch and a bit of exercise, and not be bothered by anyone or anything. After closing on the property our first task and expense was to dog proof the yard with a nice aluminum fence to the extent I felt that the day we moved in we had done him proud, and he would live his last few years with us quite contently.

Just five months after moving in, I found him one early morning lying in the lounge in a pool of blood. He had tried to chew a cancerous growth that was growing in his tail, so we rushed him over to the veterinary hospital when just one hour later the vet phoned us with the awful news that the only humane thing to do was for him to be put down. Just three days later, our daughter, Hannah, accompanied her mum and me to pay our respects and witness the process and his passing—not a dry eye between the three of us as we said our goodbyes.

To this day, I never really got over his loss, and we all miss him terribly.

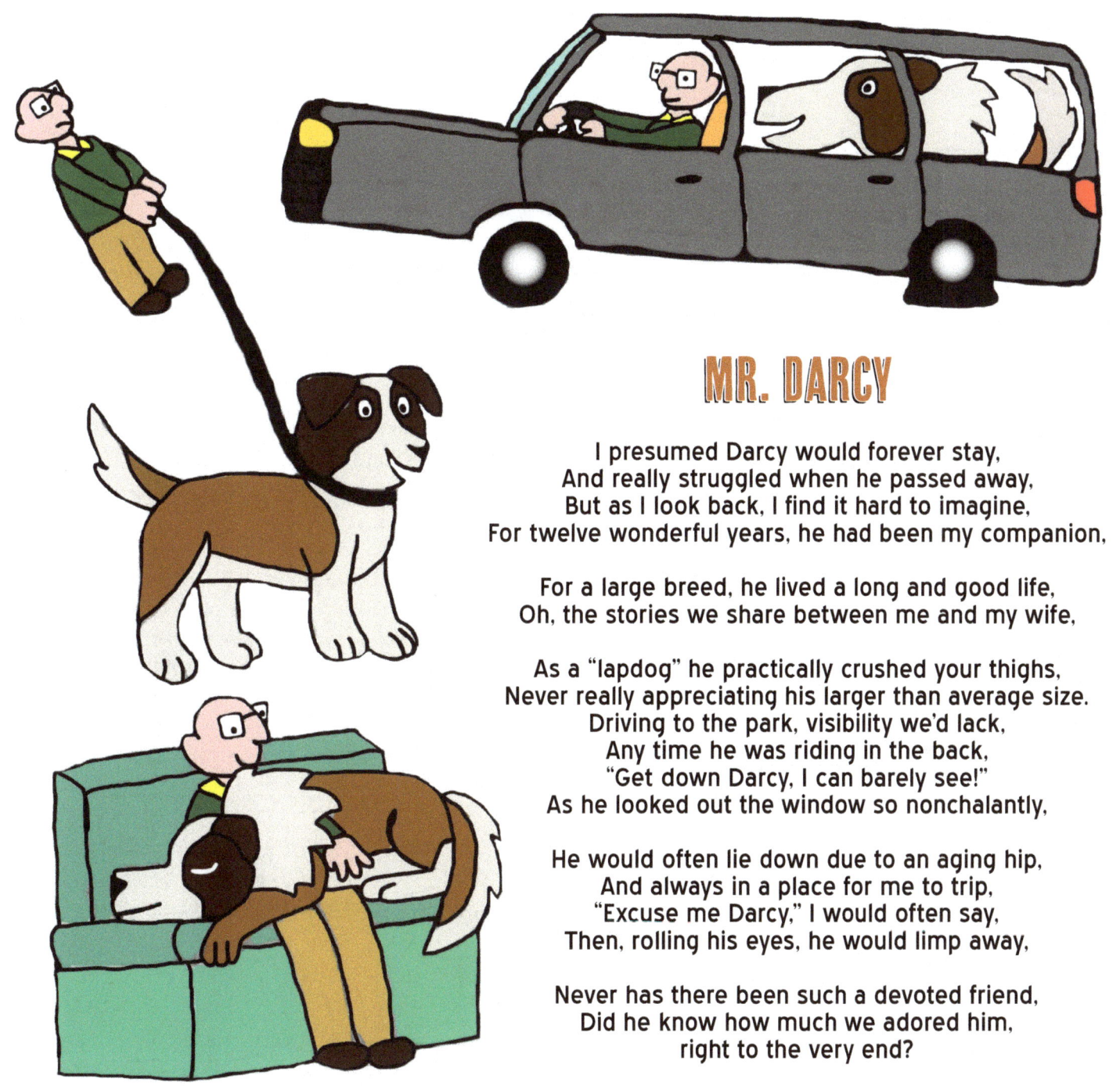

MR. DARCY

I presumed Darcy would forever stay,
And really struggled when he passed away,
But as I look back, I find it hard to imagine,
For twelve wonderful years, he had been my companion,

For a large breed, he lived a long and good life,
Oh, the stories we share between me and my wife,

As a "lapdog" he practically crushed your thighs,
Never really appreciating his larger than average size.
Driving to the park, visibility we'd lack,
Any time he was riding in the back,
"Get down Darcy, I can barely see!"
As he looked out the window so nonchalantly,

He would often lie down due to an aging hip,
And always in a place for me to trip,
"Excuse me Darcy," I would often say,
Then, rolling his eyes, he would limp away,

Never has there been such a devoted friend,
Did he know how much we adored him,
right to the very end?

24. HELLHOUND

Continuing the "doggy" theme a little while longer, the loss of Darcy left a pretty huge hole in our lives although like most things, you learn to adjust and make do. Even though I did feel Darcy was the best dog we ever had (and the best of all dogs), he could still molt in the spring and fall seasons, he could "slobber" a bit (quite a lot, actually), in short; he still needed some cleaning after, his huge frame still needed feeding and with Sarah working most days, I thought it was quite a good thing that she did not have the added burden and responsibility of looking after a dog (as well as me). Accordingly and as it turned out, I was more reluctant than her to seek a replacement, besides what dog could possibly measure up to Darcy?

Clearly, I had underestimated Sarah's own need for dog companionship because on more than one occasion, she asked that we consider getting another. Following a visit to a local dog shelter we ended up with "Bazzle". To me, from the moment I met him, he would be regarded as the "ANTI-DARCY"!

I should point out that Bazzle is spelled to be phonetically accurate. We later found out that his breed is that of a Nova Scotia Duck Tolling Retriever, a "duck-toller", for short, but Sarah wanted to name him after a British children's TV character, a fox that was called "Basil Brush" (Basil) but since American's pronounce the herb of the same name differently to us, she figured that the name tag should represent the sound she was after. For the life of me, I have no idea for what purpose since he won't come to you under any name you use. Through experience I have found it more appropriate to regard him as simply "Aya" (after "Aya-Tollah"), not that he responds to that one either!

Regardless, Bazzle is worthy of a mention in this book, since going from Darcy to him is like going from positive to negative, being up and then down. Pretty much like this poststroke journey; feeling euphoric at the sight of a slight movement of my left thumb one day and utter dejection the next day when you fail to repeat the feat.

HELLHOUND

It's been two long years since dear Darcy passed,
"Can we now replace him?" My wife then asked,
Pondering negatively about my desire to care,
Honoring Darcy, what dog could compare?

Two weeks later she asked again,
After 3 more times, my resistance would wane,
"You must decide," I finally conceded,
So, off to the shelter, she promptly proceeded,

Later that day, when she came home,
Escorting this "mutt-thing", all skin and bone,
Just as she says, "give him time to see",
Against the front door he decides to pee!

"Oh no!" I shout, "he is terrible."
Time would show, no doubt, he'd be unbearable,

Sly as a snake that should be in a zoo,
This bellyache, needed things to chew,

He started on my sheepskin coat,
After the sofa, came the TV remote,
The Grandkids toys, and the screen porch suite,
My wife's handbag and a toilet seat.

We then bought a cage with a lockable gate,
But the bed inside, he eventually ate.

"He's a monster, he's the hound from hell!"
... From on high, Darcy did tell.

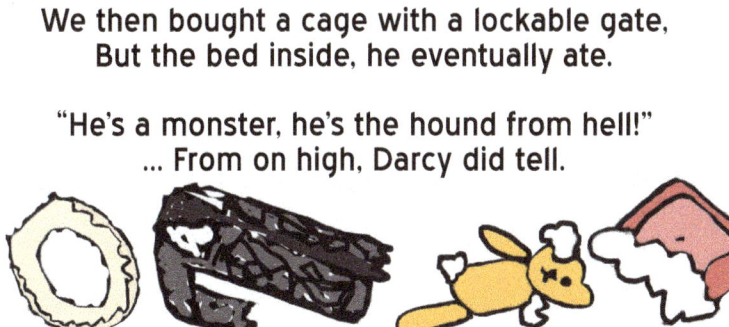
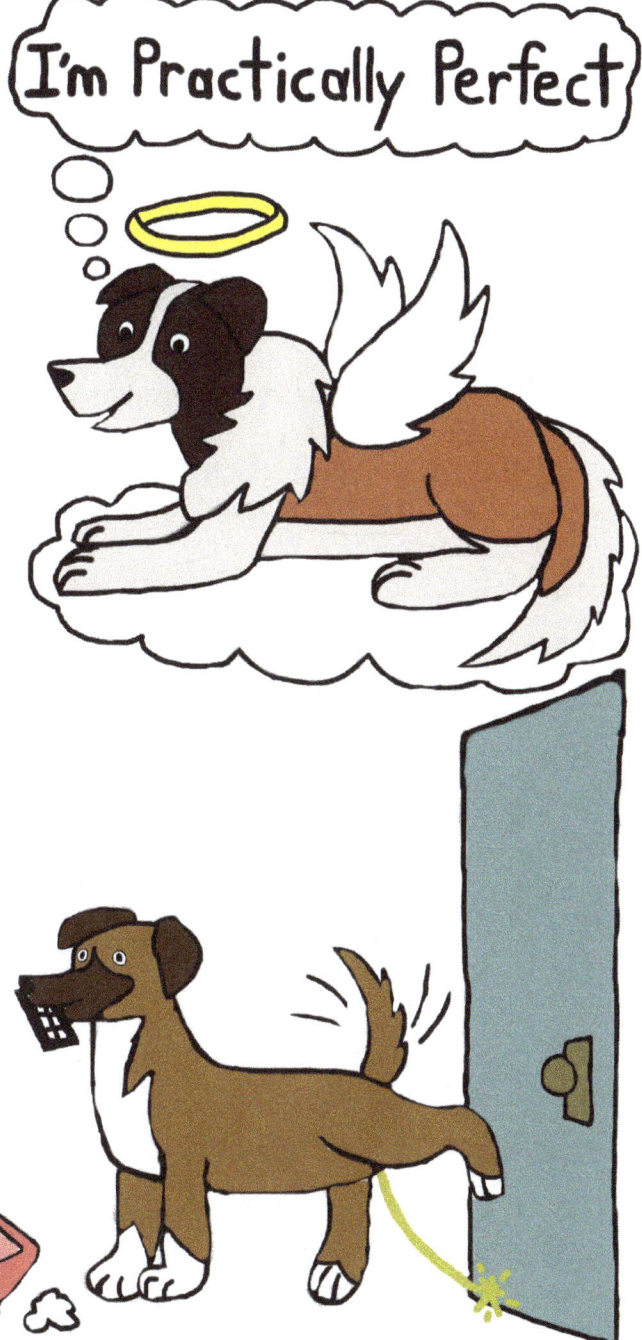

Reflections, Ramblings & Rantings of a Rancorous Stroke Survivor

25. REVERENT REFLECTION

During our Sunday service and just before we share the Lord's Prayer, our Pastor gives us a few minutes to pray alone on those matters more personal to us.

Unlike many other stroke survivors, I don't feel that my memory was unduly impacted, and on the way to church I would spend some of the time thinking about concerns close to my heart and whether it might be worth passing on some thoughts to our most Supreme Being in the hope that He might like to intervene in some positive way.

More often than not, however, during the drive home, I try to recall whether I included a particular person or concern in my prayer, so I decided to develop my own laminated "cheat card" that I could tuck away in my wallet and pull out at the appropriate time. It works for me as I believe that praying should not be reserved just for church on Sundays; I have found it handy even when sitting alone—in a doctor's waiting room, perhaps. So, this is my token effort. I do recommend it and hope it inspires you to create your own version; it helps lift me up during those dull and dreary moments and gives me a little peace and serenity along the way.

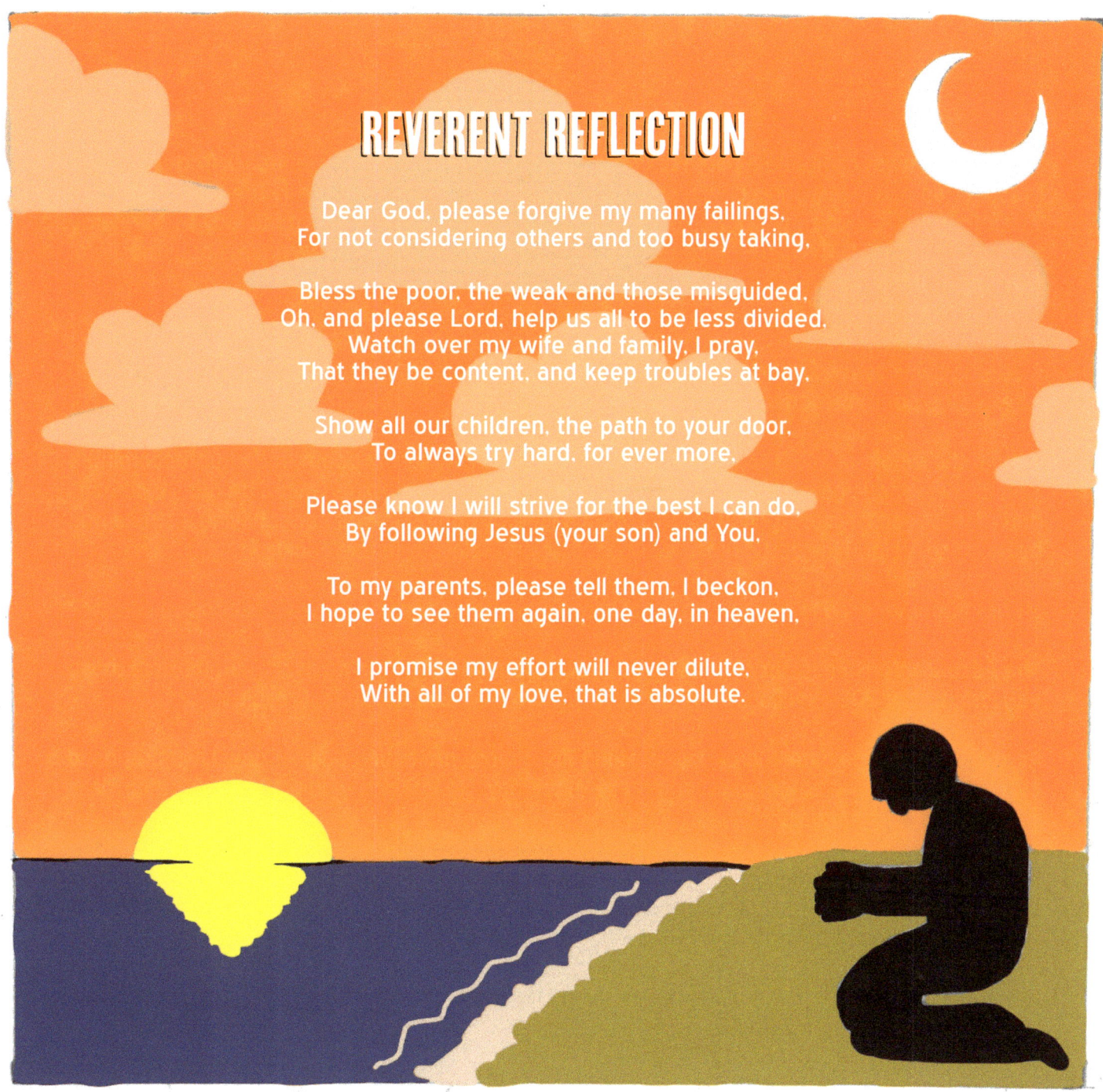

REVERENT REFLECTION

Dear God, please forgive my many failings,
For not considering others and too busy taking.

Bless the poor, the weak and those misguided,
Oh, and please Lord, help us all to be less divided.
Watch over my wife and family, I pray,
That they be content, and keep troubles at bay.

Show all our children, the path to your door,
To always try hard, for ever more.

Please know I will strive for the best I can do,
By following Jesus (your son) and You.

To my parents, please tell them, I beckon,
I hope to see them again, one day, in heaven.

I promise my effort will never dilute,
With all of my love, that is absolute.

26. WHEN IT RAINS

Every so often as I complete a poem or two, I like to try and obtain a little feedback from someone I respect and can trust their critique(s) and viewpoint. One such confide is the leader of TAP's "Back-To-Work" Group to which I belong; a talented, inspirational and charming lady by the name of Tisha Shah CCC-SLP. On one such occasion she challenged me to write a poem about the awful COVID pandemic we were all enduring at the time.

Never one for shying away from a challenge, I decided to give it a go. As you will see, the subject matter is quite generalized and fretful—despite the fact that (thankfully) I and my family (on both sides of the pond) managed to stay COVID free.

I found the whole of 2020 to be pretty depressing actually, so my poem ended up becoming a kind of metaphoric parody to the nonstop tales of woes all of us experienced on our TV screens during that year. Of course, I had to spice it up a little by adding the bit about having a stroke and by doing so, helped to keep it reasonably on topic and relevant to this book!

My grandmother used to say, "until you get some good news, the bad news just keeps on coming."

The Australian bushfires already raging from 2019 continued to create havoc right through those early months of 2020; millions of innocent animals were killed as a direct result.

At around the same time, the people of Hong Kong were protesting against new laws proposed by the Chinese government—it seemed like every day, Hong Kong would be a picture of mass protestation and tear gas.

The wrongful killing of George Floyd in May of that year was particularly distressing to all those that witnessed the injustice committed and triggered a massive round of anti-racist activity that led to serious unrest not only in America but within many countries around the world.

In short, 2020 was the worst of years and should be expunged from everybody's memory bank!

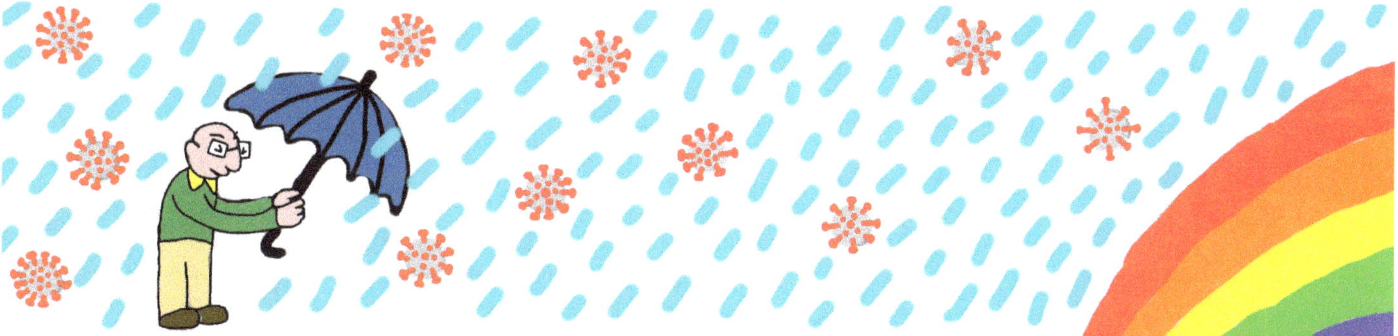

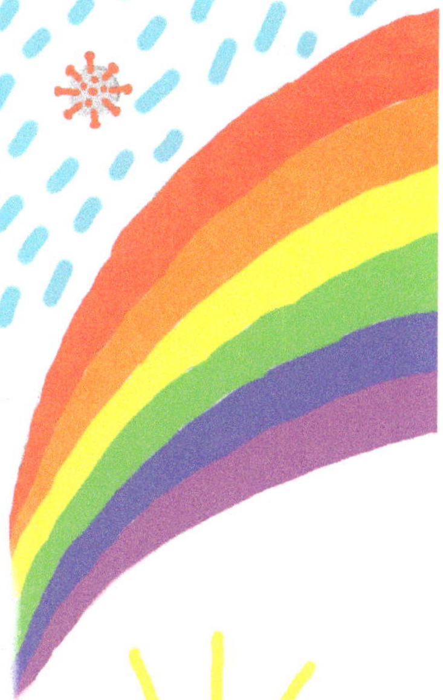

WHEN IT RAINS

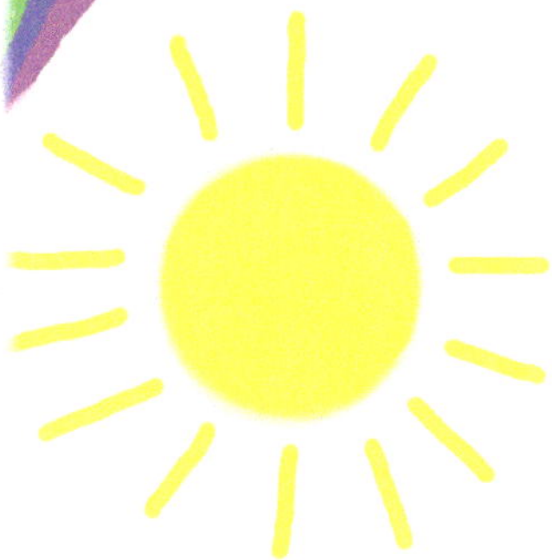

Just when you thought it couldn't get worse,
One thing after another, unable to reverse,
Convinced I was given a terrible curse,
A sinner's sentence—obliged to disburse,

The business was failing, nothing went right,
Downturn prevailing, couldn't muster the fight,
Every bank said I was not worth a loan,
My staff all left, and I was on my own,

That's when the stroke hit and left us penniless,
My best dog died, and my wife got up and left,
She said, "It's just the way it is, these things are sent to try us",
When someone I never met, gives me a virus!

There is no point in dwelling, feeling sad and forlorn,
I've no intent in telling, I wish I wasn't born,
No words expelling, hate and pouring scorn,
I'll just file it to the past and await a bright new dawn.

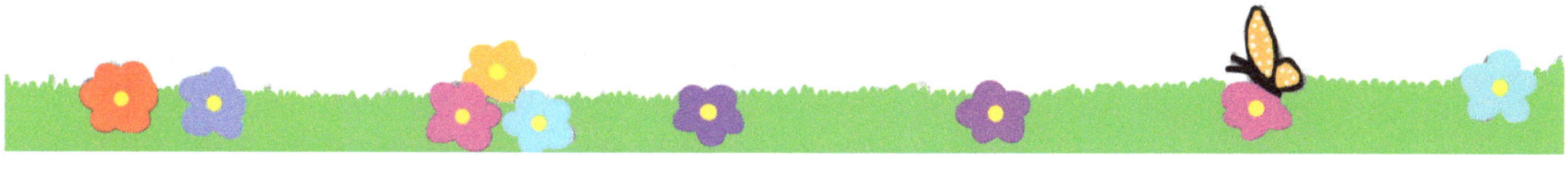

27. GRAMPSI'S LAW

It never dawned on me that one day, I could ever be a grandfather. I remember both my mum and dad's parents were really old (at least they seemed to be, to me)! Surely, I could never be that old? Or that lucky to live that long, that lucky to become a grandfather? Surely not.

It is difficult for me to express the sheer excitement and joy that came over me the moment I was told that we were expecting our first grandchild and barely two years had passed when we were greeted with another. Heck, how lucky we are!

I am very proud of our three children and how they turned out. Mainly thanks to my wife, Sarah, who kept their noses clean and supported their various endeavors—It seemed I was always too busy most of the time to take any credit. At least now I have an opportunity to play a positive role with my grandchildren.

The good news about having a stroke, is that I have way more time to show interest in my grandchildren's pursuits, the bad news about having a stroke is that I don't think I would be very good chasing a soccer ball in the yard or climbing a tree!

That said, I am more than capable of talking with them and showing interest in their various endeavors.

The simple act of writing down my (good faith) intentions and posting on my office wall as a daily reminder improves the odds of me doing my bit, I feel.

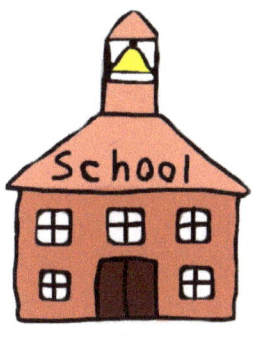
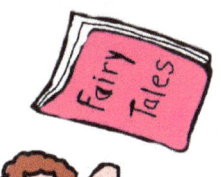
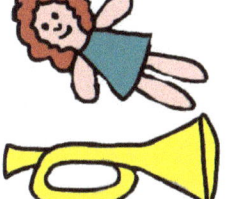
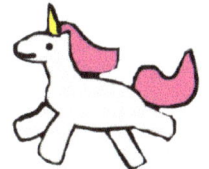
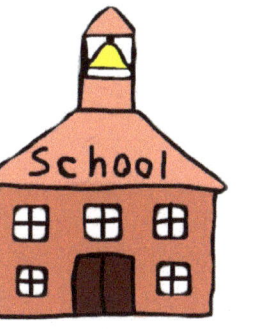
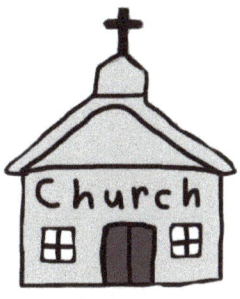
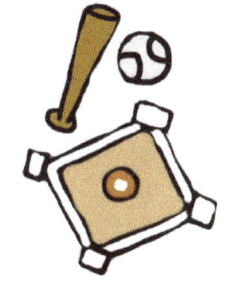
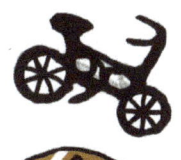
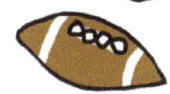

GRAMPSI'S LAW

Being a grandfather is a chore I take seriously,
A mission I'll adore deliriously,
Passing on the values that were passed down to me,
By both my grandfathers, so conscientiously.

I shall help them with their building blocks,
Show excitement unwrapping my birthday socks,

Always portray the perfect Gent,
And cheer them on at their school event,

When they are down, I will offer smiles and comfort,
And be the first to praise when they are triumphant,

I will sit with them happily in the afternoon,
And try not to snore during their favorite cartoon,

These things I promise from the bottom of my heart,
To help give their life's journey, the best possible start.

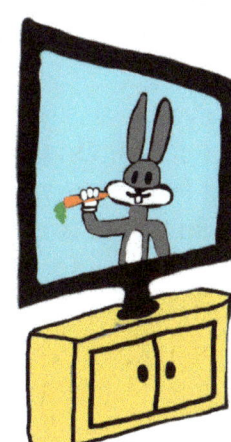
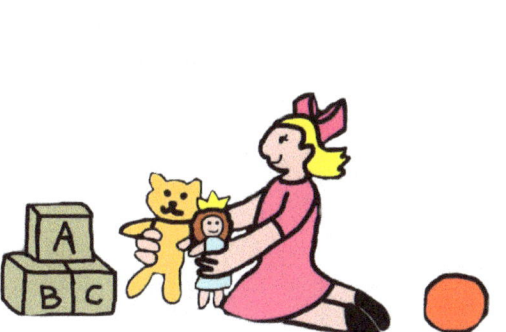
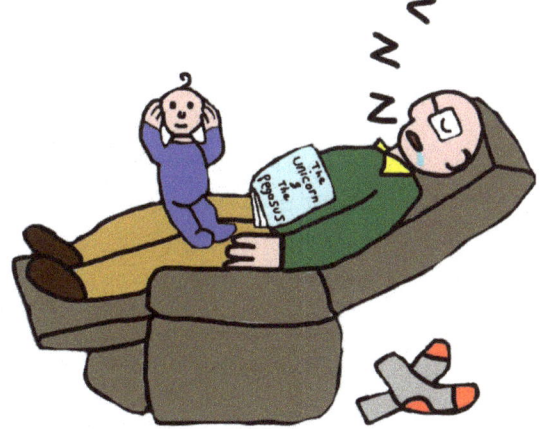

Reflections, Ramblings & Rantings of a Rancorous Stroke Survivor

28. CAVALRY OF THE CLOUDS

My (maternal) grandfather, (Grandpa) Thomas Henry Swann (1899-1982) saw action in both world wars; as with so many of his generation, he left home at sixteen years old very keen to enlist in the army.

Between the years 1977-1980, Grandpa was transferred to a specialist chest hospital in the county of Kent in the southeast of England and quite local to my parents' home which gave my girlfriend at the time, Sarah, and me the opportunity to undertake the forty minute motorbike ride to visit with him on the occasional weekend. Many a precious moment was gained when we had the opportunity to wheel him out into the garden on a nice sunny day and hear stories about his past and some of his wartime experiences...

In the Great War, it was bad enough being situated close to the front line always in sight and shooting range of a formidable foe, but considering the miserable weather and living conditions in the trenches—damp, mud, gas, rats, and lice, it was quite understandable that when the army created a new branch called the Royal Flying Corps (RFC), that would later become the Royal Air Force (RAF), and were looking for volunteers to join, Grandpa and many others were very quick to apply.

The term, "Cavalry of the clouds" used to describe the RFC was first coined by David Lloyd George, Britain's prime minister (1916-1922) in a speech to the House of Commons in October 1917.

Despite George's attempt to "glamorize" the role of airmen, in those early days, it was a highly risky occupation with untested, often unreliable technology and coupled with minimal training, the average life expectancy of a WW1 airman was barely 69 flying hours! Parachutes, whilst recently invented, were not standard issue back then—apparently those higher up the chain of command needed the planes back (in any condition) and did not wish to encourage air crew to jump over the side if they got into difficulty.

The RFC's first priority was to undertake reconnaissance and provide necessary intelligence relating to enemy troop and armament movement, new trench construction and other useful tactical information to the army on the ground. Previously, this data was provided by "observers" in some kind of tethered balloon—highly vulnerable to enemy fire, but within a couple of years, reconnaissance balloons were superseded by "heavier than air" (and more nimble) flying machines which allowed their role to expand to more offensive duties (like bombing raids).Thomas Henry successfully applied to become an "observer" holding the rank of second lieutenant—in most aircraft of the time, this was the guy that would sit in the back of the plane responsible for operating the side mounted camera; also at his disposal, were a couple of bombs straddled to each wing and a Lewis machine gun behind his seat to fend off enemy fighter planes.

On one occasion, Grandpa told us the story of (and wanted to pay tribute to) the heroic actions of his pilot, Captain Patrick Eliot Welchman (1895-1918) when on a raid to support ground troops in the North of France (behind the front line) in September 1918, happened across a greater number of enemy planes. The ensuing dogfight had Grandpa shot in the back of the leg and despite being severely wounded in the chest and wrestling the controls, Captain Welchman managed to guide the damaged aircraft onto a farmer's field safely below. They were both captured and became prisoners of war. Grandpa was eventually released and repatriated on November 26th, 1918, but Captain Welchman was not so fortunate—having died from "neglect of wounds" on November 29, 1918 just two weeks following Armistice Day (cessation of fighting on the Western Front). There was absolutely no doubt in Grandpa's mind, that Captain Patrick Welchman saved his life that day on September 26, 1918.

During his time in captivity, Grandpa kept thinking about his friends in the mess hall each evening and wondered whether they would undertake the traditional toast to the two empty chairs they used to occupy or whether the squadron managed to fill them with other unsuspecting dreamers as was often the case when airmen failed to return home.

The following poem is my very small tribute to Captain Welchman, my grandpa and the many heroes of their generation that signed up for military service for the benefit of us all.

I like to think that stroke survivors have a little of that "adventurous spirit" as they embark on their journey knowing very little of what might lie in store, but always with the hope (and belief) that all will be alright in the end.

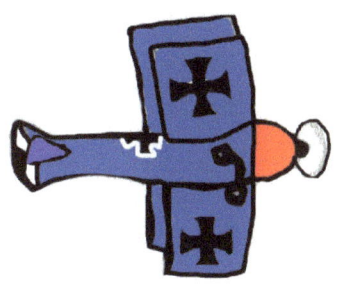
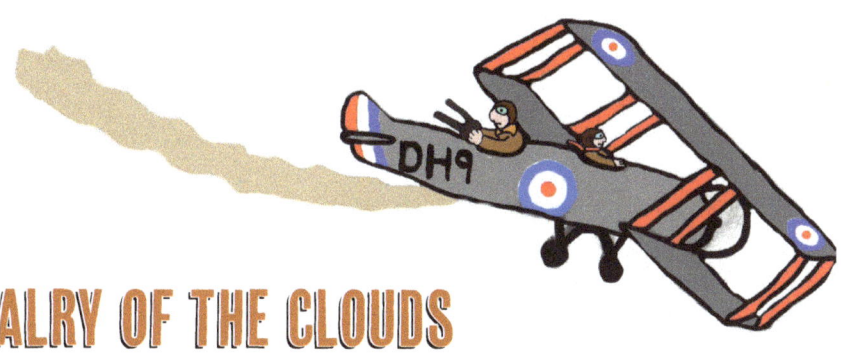

CAVALRY OF THE CLOUDS

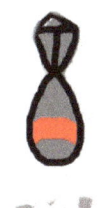
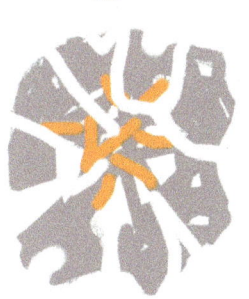

Sleeping with rats in this dark, damp, dingy trench,
Cordite and death give the air its stench,
Tomorrow will come, and we will do it again,
My mates and me, most foolish of men.

"Over the top, soon" our colonel said,
Lives cut short, forever living in dread,
Distracted by sounds from overhead.

"Lucky Blighters!" an earnest sigh,
Far from here, up there in the sky,
If only... I could fly,
Must take the opportunity to apply.

Six in the morn', we will be in the air,
It will be cold at dawn, but colder up there,
We will hide in the sun, so foes beware,
Doing our best, doing our share.

Mission underway, diminishing cares,
Just silly pawns, remembered by chairs.

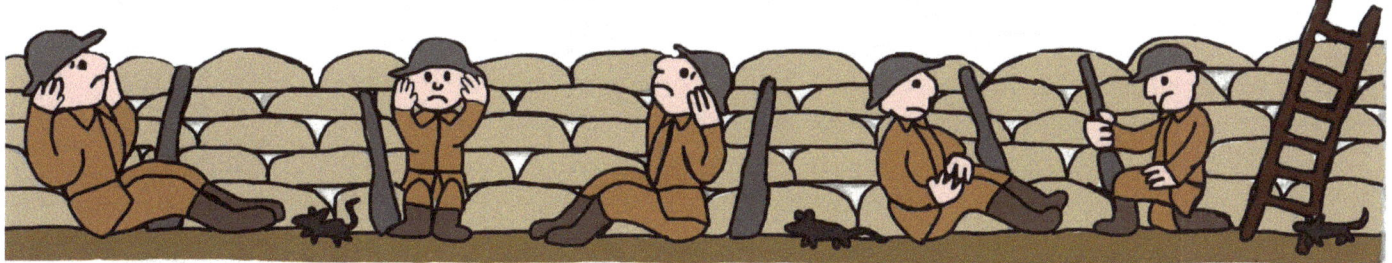

29. YOUNG AT HEART

At the time of Thomas Henry's death, his wife of 55 years, Marjorie (Madge) Swann (1905-1988) (my Nan) would have been 77 years old. When she passed away 6 years later, my mother came across a card with a hand-written poem alongside a self-portrait amongst her personal effects that I feel, summed up the lady perfectly.

Nan was born and raised in the county of Yorkshire in the north of England, and she had a truly wicked (Yorkshire) sense of humor.

She was a trained Seamstress and spent a couple of months making my wife, Sarah's wedding dress for our big day—a beautiful result and saved us a small fortune.

As young grandchildren, we grew up convinced that Grandpa was shot in the buttock because (according to her) during the first world war, he got so fed up one day, he climbed out of his trench shouted over to the German line, "Oy, you lot!" then proceeded to pull down his trousers and underwear adding, "this is what I think of you!" giving them a full 'mooning' gesture, "and they shot him, they did, right in the bum!" , "bloody fool, never been able to sit still since", she would add.

It was in fact my Nan's version of Grandpa's war wound that allowed me to eventually extract the truth in his later years, "so Grandpa, tell us how you really got shot in the bottom?" I asked and it was then that he told us it wasn't a trench incident at all but rather when he was flying with the RFC, further, he was not shot in the buttock area at all, he was wounded in the Gluteus at the back side and top of his leg. Resulting from being shot from behind in a dogfight.

It's only right having extolled the virtues of my grandfather earlier that I include a reference to my Nan here; and her (original, hand-written) version of how she thought of herself; I think, is far better than I could possibly convey graphically.

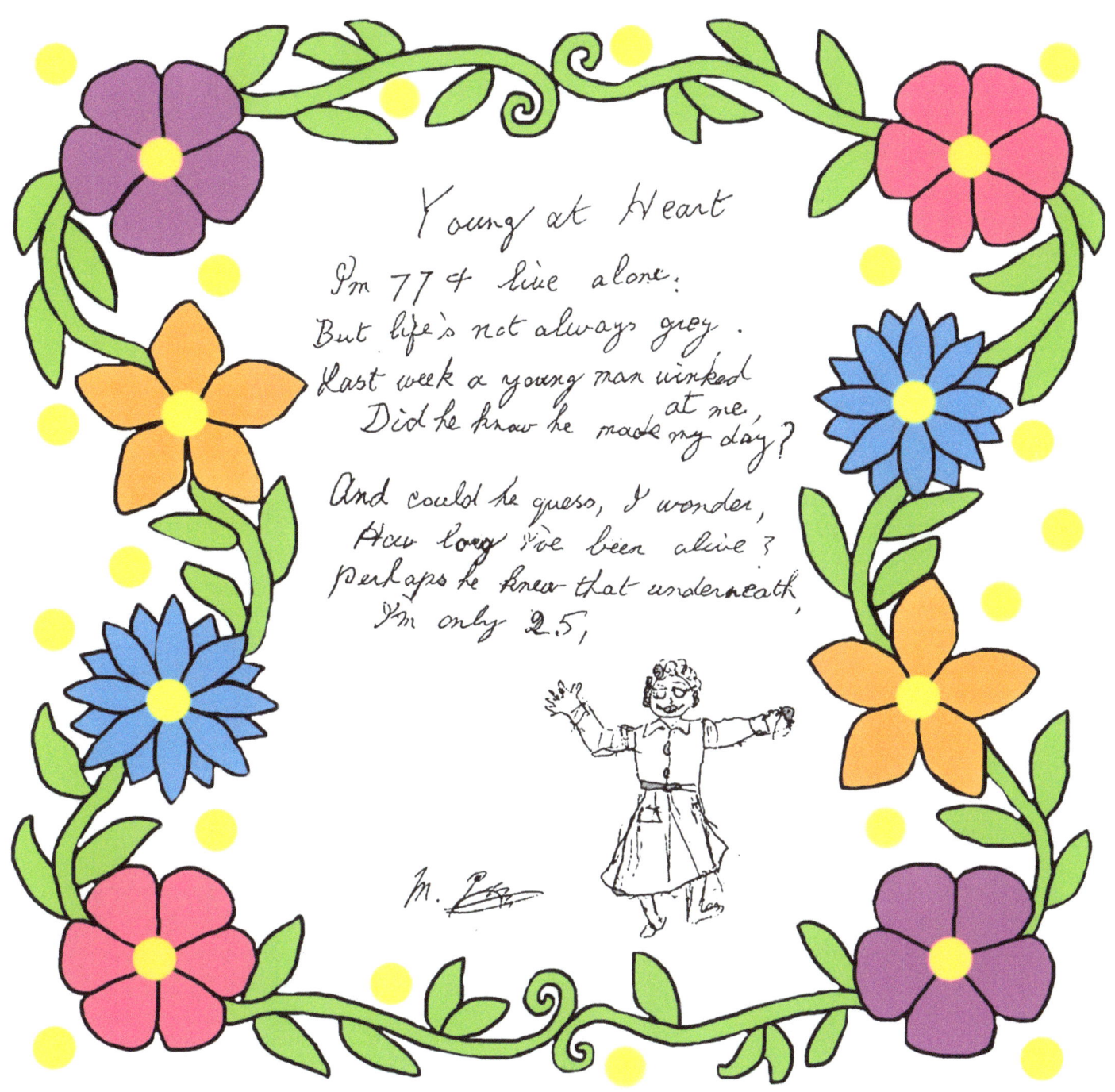

Young at Heart

I'm 77 & live alone:
But life's not always grey.
Last week a young man winked at me,
  Did he know he made my day?

And could he guess, I wonder,
  How long I've been alive?
Perhaps he knew that underneath,
I'm only 25.

30. FAIREST OF LADIES

I am not ashamed to admit that I have been in love with another woman for a very long time—even at the time of proposing to my wife, Sarah, many years ago! My only solace is knowing that she has known the truth for many years, and I think her acceptance of my obsession is largely down to me knowing of her adoration, in almost equal measure, of Robert Redford for about the same time, and he is still alive!!

I was about twelve years old when I first saw Audrey Hepburn. My parents loved musicals and when television started screening some of the old classics, I and my siblings were obliged to watch. My Fair Lady (1953) was one of those hits from the past (winning 8 Oscars) and capitalized on the stardom she earned from her first top billing (Oscar winning) role in Roman Holiday around ten years earlier. The movie was in color and truly captured her elegance and charm with the fabulous wardrobe she wore from a lowly, poor Cockney flower girl to when she mingles with members of the aristocracy by the end and climax of the picture. As directors and producers would later testify, the camera absolutely loved her, as did I. A long and successful collaboration with Hubert de Givenchy helped immortalize her as a fashion icon for all ages.

Audrey's last top billing role was in the movie, Robin and Marian (starring alongside Sean Connery) in 1976, she was now forty-seven years old and still looking and performing to perfection.

Her love for children alongside her personal experiences (malnourished when growing up in Nazi occupied Holland) compelled her to accept the invitation to become a full-time ambassador for UNICEF during the late 1980s where she spent much of her time highlighting the plight of starving children in Africa, Asia, and Latin America and where she was often seen conversing in the six different languages she spoke fluently with the world's media outlets only taking the occasional break for a (smaller, cameo type) movie role. She devoted a huge amount of her time to this charitable work tirelessly visible on the front line. She could be seen amongst the poor and starving children of the third world(s).

I think it was through witnessing, first-hand, the many selfless acts of work during this poststroke journey that reminded me and rekindled my fondness of her. From the nurses in the hospitals to the therapists in the outpatient clinics and to all those dedicated professionals that give up so much of their time to organize and run the stroke support groups I attend and benefit from. It is understandable that Audrey's background allowed her to be empathetic and helped fuel her charitable nature, but I have often wondered what is that magic ingredient that has encouraged others to show similar levels of compassion and giving; I wonder, what was behind their calling?

I last saw Audrey Hepburn receiving a special (outstanding contribution) award at the 1992 BAFTA's (British equivalent of the Oscars). The physically measured and gracefully long curtsey she performed in front of Princess Anne and the charm and generosity of her acceptance speech belied the colon cancer that had snuck up on her. Just ten months later at the age of (only) 63 in January 1993 she died, surrounded by her loved ones at her home in Switzerland. A great and full life run and the passing of a legend without equal—then or since, in my opinion.

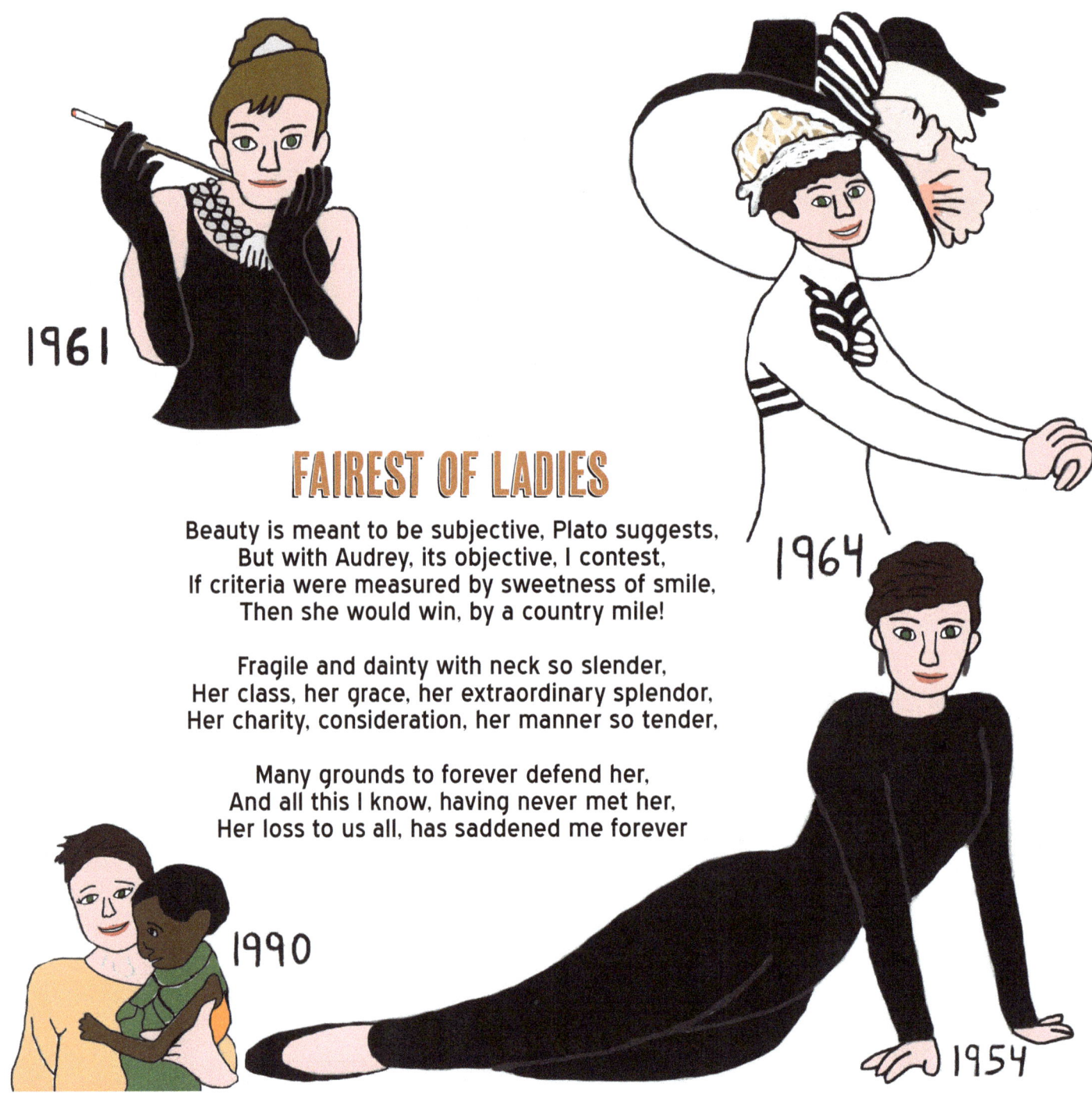

FAIREST OF LADIES

Beauty is meant to be subjective, Plato suggests,
But with Audrey, its objective, I contest,
If criteria were measured by sweetness of smile,
Then she would win, by a country mile!

Fragile and dainty with neck so slender,
Her class, her grace, her extraordinary splendor,
Her charity, consideration, her manner so tender,

Many grounds to forever defend her,
And all this I know, having never met her,
Her loss to us all, has saddened me forever

BAD RHYMES, NO REASON

31. BETTER THAN THE REST

As I read books on stroke survival and hear from others within the stroke community, the love and support afforded to a stroke survivor from friends and particularly family members, cannot be understated. Such was the case when my dear old mother arrived in North Carolina for my son's wedding celebrations which coincided within two days of my stroke event. She was one of the first to see me in hospital and during those early years she was always available at the end of the phone to give me that proverbial "kick" needed to remind me that compared to many, I was really quite lucky and doing pretty well. Although she is no longer here physically, I sense her presence and guidance in many of my daily activities. I continue to strive in the hope that I can make her proud one day.

And so, continuing this short theme of poems to extraordinary women of my life, I must pay homage to mum, June Pamela Barton (1931-2018). I was so proud of her, a highly accomplished lady that gave up a promising career in Haute Couture (a gift she inherited from her mother) so that she could stay at home and devote a great deal of time to raising her four children along with supporting her husband's demanding business activities. Despite contracting cancer in her early 60s she became an established (watercolor) artist and was teaching classes in both North Carolina and England up until six months before the cancer took her away from us at the age of 87.

June Pamela Barton (1931-2018)

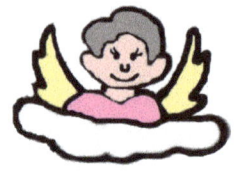

BETTER THAN THE REST

Today marks a year since she passed away,
She remains on my mind, every single day,
Her influence on me, I cannot understate,
To see her once more, I can barely wait,

I know she's up there, looking down,
Continuing to inspire me, and make her proud,

Everybody thinks their mother is best,
Sorry, but mine will forever be, better than the rest!

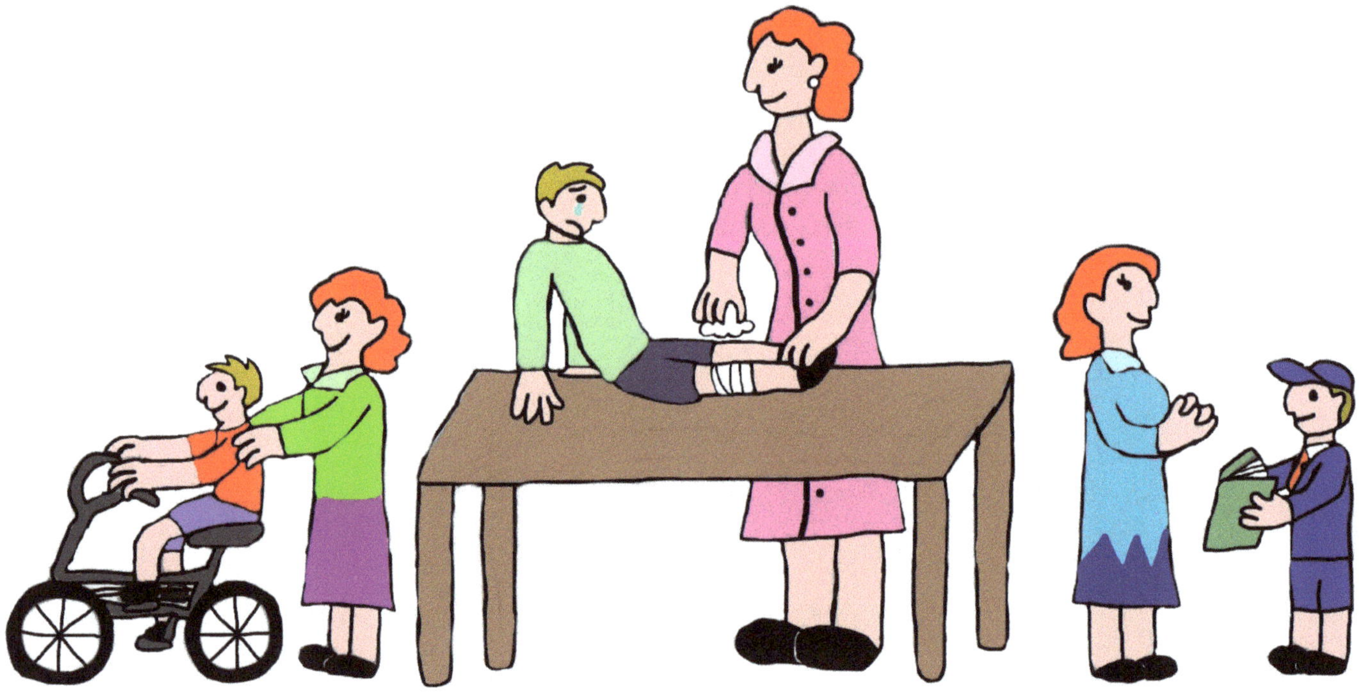

32. TROUBLE AND STRIFE

For those not familiar with London's Cockney Rhyming Slang, "dog and bone" means "phone"; "elephant's trunk" means "drunk"; "charlie pride" means "ride" so putting it together, one guy could say to another … "So there I was, elephant's trunk, got on the dog and bone called trouble and said I needed a charlie! "Trouble" comes from "trouble and strife", which of course, means "wife", which in my case, means Sarah.

Goodness, didn't I do well? Considering my life as a whole, my single best achievement was marrying this lady back in 1983. I am not sure she could say the same, but for some reason, she has stood by my side these years despite my many faults and flaws, and I love her to bits!

Sarah never signed up to be a caregiver, other than some pre-college part-time work in a pharmacy; she has had no formal medical training although her schooling in ancient Greek and Latin has helped greatly to understanding the cocktail of medications I have been obliged to take over the years. But as with me, the stroke was a major shock with a sudden need to learn, understand, and adapt to a foreign situation and by Jove, she more than rose to the challenge.

With the loss of our primary income, the moment she became comfortable with my ability to fend for myself around the house, she would work any overtime available to help make up the difference. Around the time of the event, she was contemplating her retirement from work in the hope that her 401K pension could meet her needs. The only regret ever expressed was from my end, not hers. She was a trooper promoted to a general and as I have become more self-sufficient, she has not been so proud to shy away from rank of sergeant major—consistently rallying and motivating her one soldier (me) to do his best.

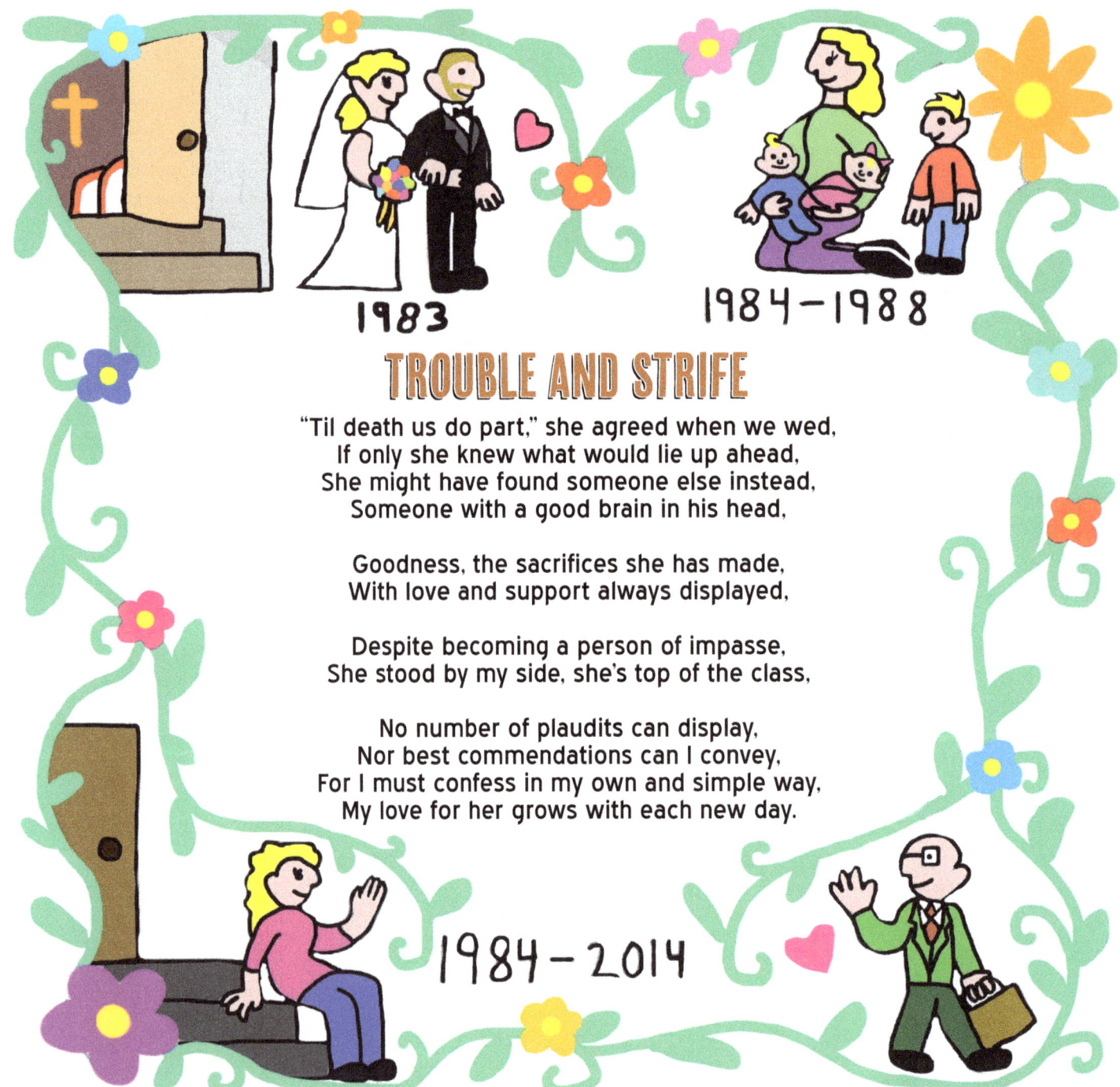

TROUBLE AND STRIFE

"Til death us do part," she agreed when we wed,
If only she knew what would lie up ahead,
She might have found someone else instead,
Someone with a good brain in his head,

Goodness, the sacrifices she has made,
With love and support always displayed,

Despite becoming a person of impasse,
She stood by my side, she's top of the class,

No number of plaudits can display,
Nor best commendations can I convey,
For I must confess in my own and simple way,
My love for her grows with each new day.

33. SOMETHING

For some time now, I have been struggling a little with the merits of my (almost) blind acceptance of the poststroke condition(s) I have—my disabilities and limitations etc., on the basis that whilst I have become happier and more content with my new self (along with impairments) and making do as best I can with what I have, I am aware that in doing so, I have lost some of the desire required to improve further. That said, I did wake up one morning last year with something of a "what the heck, buck your ideas up" attitude and wanted to make a bit more of an effort to the extent that I should consider an alternative approach since after six years of the more conventional therapies, I had made little to no progress. Indeed, since being told I was wasting my time because "there was no functional improvement", I had not seen a qualified PT (or OT) in over twelve months.

I sought out a specialist practitioner in the area of occupational therapy based in California as someone that had helped people with similar physical disabilities to me, but over a shorter and more intensive (five day) therapy session period. This adventure was not something I could obtain through our regular medical insurance, and it was not going to be cheap, but upon the passing of my mother, her reasonable estate left me enough money that helped defray the expense.

He accepted my application and after completing the necessary questionnaires and obtaining the correct (negative) COVID test result, Sarah and I booked our flights and accommodation and so we headed off to the West Coast.

Just witnessing my walk to the therapy table on our first meeting confirmed to him the sorry state I was in. Until that time, I was quite pleased with myself; first, that I was reasonably mobile and second, that I undertook a twenty-minute walk in the early hours of each and every morning for the past one and a half years. But apparently, from what I understood, my walking technique was so bad that it had a consequential and negative affect on my overall posture that contributed to much of the continued dysfunction and spasticity within my arm and hand—something that upon reviewing a video my son took quite recently, my very first (outpatient) PT, Katie, warned me about, another example of my inability to listen to the right advice when given.

He made me no promises about the level of restoration he could do for me other than it would be an ongoing process, extending long after I leave his clinic, five days later.

In my case, the stroke to the right side of my brain has resulted much more in a physical disability (to my left side limbs) than a cognitive one, and although I have some communication and organizational issues to contend with, compared to many, these are relatively minor. "Hemiplegia" is the medical term for my physical condition and is defined as "muscle weakness and partial paralysis to one side of the body". It has been very difficult for me to deal with and even harder to define, I am led to believe it is incurable, but with continued stretching and therapy the effects can be alleviated to some degree.

Ever since leaving the hospital the remnant spasticity causes my arm to bend at the elbow with my hand (totally locked closed) residing near my belly button.

Whilst I recognize the importance, as emphasized by the professional therapist, that goal setting as a tool plays for the speedy recovery process of the stroke survivor, I found that in my case, the definition of a reasonable goal was in itself, a target too far. And an unreasonable goal only led to frustration and disappointment when I failed to realize it.

After ten three-hour (quite grueling) sessions, when I left his clinic, I had learned a new and better walking technique along with some new stretching exercises and my arm was significantly looser than it had ever been. With the purchase of a special WHO device (Wrist-Hand Orthotic) which I wear most days of the week, five months later, my arm now hangs by my side much more naturally than it has ever been in the past seven and a half years. My hand is equally loose and almost open. No question, I am much better than I was and very much looking forward to signing up for another course of treatment quite soon. Little by little, bit by bit, one step at a time, I guess.

The following poem is my clumsy attempt to express my personal and ongoing experience(s) of dealing with hemiplegia over the years, but still, I am not convinced that the reader can truly appreciate what it really means and the utter demoralization that nearly two percent of the population with some form of paralysis experiences mentally, every day.

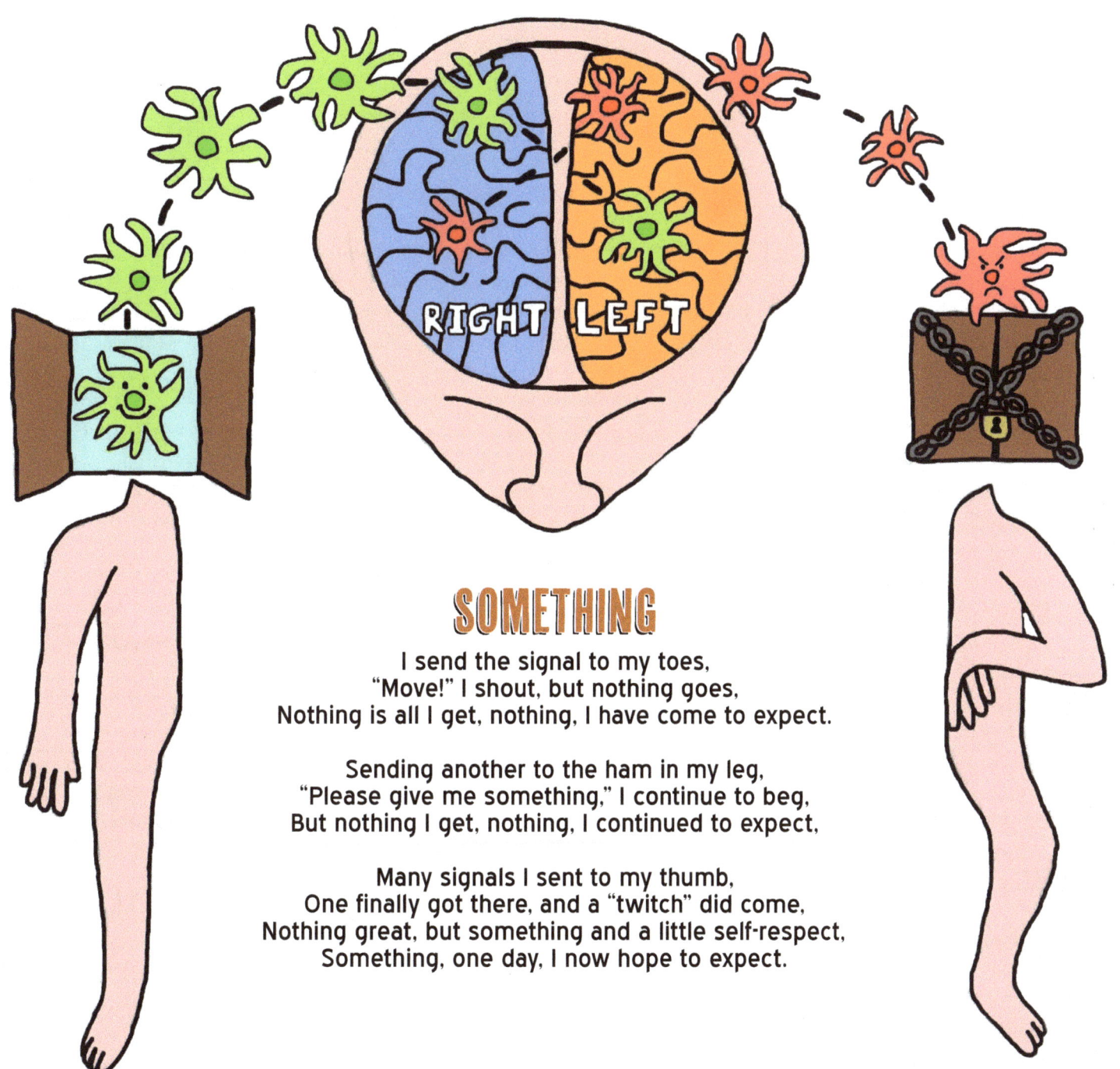

SOMETHING

I send the signal to my toes,
"Move!" I shout, but nothing goes,
Nothing is all I get, nothing, I have come to expect.

Sending another to the ham in my leg,
"Please give me something," I continue to beg,
But nothing I get, nothing, I continued to expect,

Many signals I sent to my thumb,
One finally got there, and a "twitch" did come,
Nothing great, but something and a little self-respect,
Something, one day, I now hope to expect.

34. WIND IN MY SAILS

When I was around ten years old, my father sent me away on a group sailing course—it was quite basic and we learned elementary navigation theory along with simple maneuvering of a small sailboat, that sort of thing. I remember the boat provided for training was known as an "International-420" sailing dinghy, a single mast with two sails (main and jib), quite small (<14 ft) and the sort of vessel that could be managed singlehandedly by a young lad, as I was then. From there, I got the sailing bug and future vacations by the seaside would have me renting out a sailboat which was fine when it was just me or me and my wife. Then the kids came along, and it was never practical to take out a small sailboat with all five of us in it. One year, with a little encouragement from a good friend, Sarah and I decided to go down to Florida and undertake a course to earn our ASA-104 Captain's licenses which would then allow us to rent and sail much bigger yachts where we could take the whole family to the mild climate and crystal waters of the Caribbean Islands, for example. We did this for a couple of years and like many things, wondered why we had not done it sooner! We have been back to the Caribbean many times and had some very special and wonderful trips.

Then the stroke came, and it seemed an impossible dream to do it once more. An English friend of mine, Simon Bishop, with a similar background and love for sailing as me invited us to join him and his wife Gilly, to regain "my sea-legs". When I told Katie Stephens PT, NCS, my first physical therapist (responsible for getting me out of the wheelchair initially), she too felt that I could do it—with a little hard work and preparation, of course. Accordingly on my next visit to her clinic, she went to great lengths setting up a bunch of obstacles designed in such a way to act as a "man-overboard" situation with the purpose and challenge of me getting back onto a boat using only my one (functional) side of my body. At the time, we were living in our first (US) house which had a swimming pool in the yard and between therapies and a daily (ugly looking) swim, I was ready, so off we went!

It was just ten days onboard a very nice three cabin, 46 ft cruising catamaran, again sailing around the British Virgin Islands which is quite an easy sail and with the added benefit of my friend Simon undertaking most of the captain's responsibilities, it could not be better and less troublesome than I had initially feared.

One evening, I volunteered to cook the party a simple barbecue on a small charcoal grill that was secured to a railing located at the stern (rear) of the vessel. With my wife handing me the food (wings and sausages etc.), I had a small torch (flashlight) between my teeth allowing my good hand to be free for basting and flipping the meat, I was really quite content standing and balancing behind the grill and doing my bit; that was until a passing speedboat caused a sizeable wake making ours "bounce" and unable to grab a supporting railing, I fell backwards into the water! The concerned onlookers immediately got to their feet and inquired, "are you okay?" and as I tried to say "fine" the torch left my mouth and snaked its way slowly down to the seabed— fortunately with the light still shining it settled right next to the barbecue tongs that I also dropped in my pathetic attempt to save myself.

The good news was that through Katie's training and preparation, I managed to side stroke back to the boat and get myself back in. My captain friend was the only other to get wet that evening since he quickly dived in to retrieve the flashlight and tongs—so that we could salvage the overly "charred" food and try to enjoy our meal.

Sailing is such a great activity to enjoy—the stars at night are never brighter than when you are on the water in the middle of nowhere. With no deadlines to meet, you can enjoy the sound of the water sloshing against the hull and the breeze filling the sails. It is the perfect time to totally relax and get your thoughts together.

Most of us are descendants of sailors and indeed so much of our everyday expressions come from our ancestors past nautical terms that all too often seem so relevant to our lives today.

Despite the advancements I have made during my recovery journey, there have been many occasions when I have felt "all at sea" and with the absence of progression, sometimes, the "wind has been taken out of my sails" rendering me "dead in the water". The following poem, however, I hope (and feel), mirrors my journey, concluding on a more positive note.

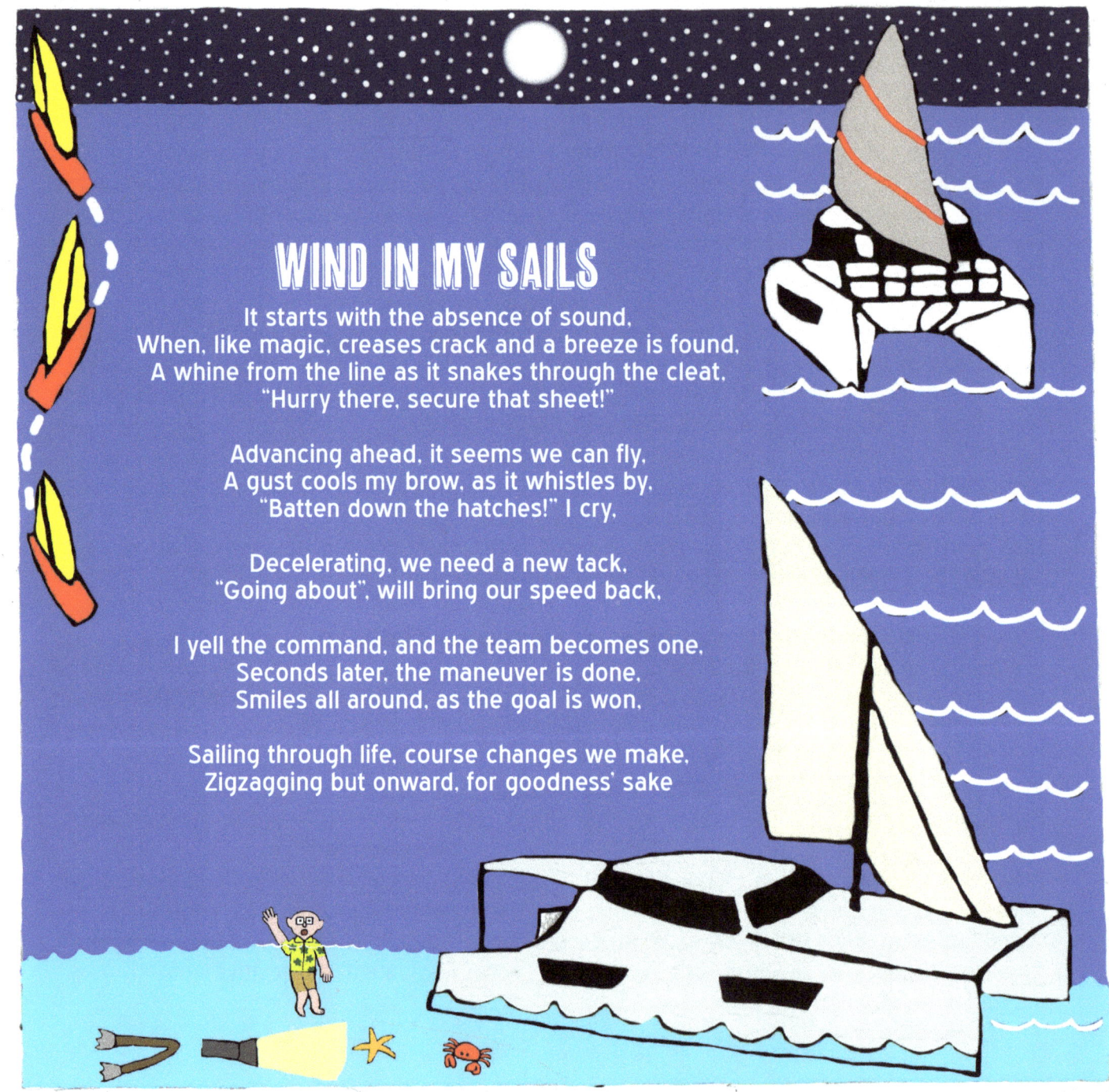

WIND IN MY SAILS

It starts with the absence of sound,
When, like magic, creases crack and a breeze is found,
A whine from the line as it snakes through the cleat,
"Hurry there, secure that sheet!"

Advancing ahead, it seems we can fly,
A gust cools my brow, as it whistles by,
"Batten down the hatches!" I cry.

Decelerating, we need a new tack,
"Going about", will bring our speed back,

I yell the command, and the team becomes one,
Seconds later, the maneuver is done,
Smiles all around, as the goal is won,

Sailing through life, course changes we make,
Zigzagging but onward, for goodness' sake

BAD RHYMES, NO REASON

35. NEUROPLASTICITY

Of all the organs and muscles in the human body the brain demands the most oxygen. If the oxygen supply is cut off for just five minutes, brain cells will begin to die, irrevocably! And this is what happens during a stroke event either by "Ischemic" (a blockage of blood supply) or by "hemorrhagic" (a rupture or loss of blood supply). Within those brain cells are neurons and these are the important cells that need the oxygen the most and through they are designed transmit and carry information within the brain and from there, to other parts of the body. Dead neurons cannot be rescued or repaired; sadly, therefore the damaged area of the brain can never function as it did before the injury.

That said, over recent years, neuroscientific research has found that the brain, regardless of age, is "plastic" and capable of "rewiring" itself. An SLP acquaintance of mine best explained it likening the brain as a map made up of roads for the millions of microscopic neurons in their miniature vehicles to travel with their little pieces of information that they need to deliver and when there is major roadwork (like a giant sinkhole) they learn to detour and find an alternative route to their destination. As stroke survivors, the more we work the brain and try to send signals—however hard it may be, then the better the outcome. I think it is this single phenomenon that has given me the best hope for returning to productive living sometime in the future.

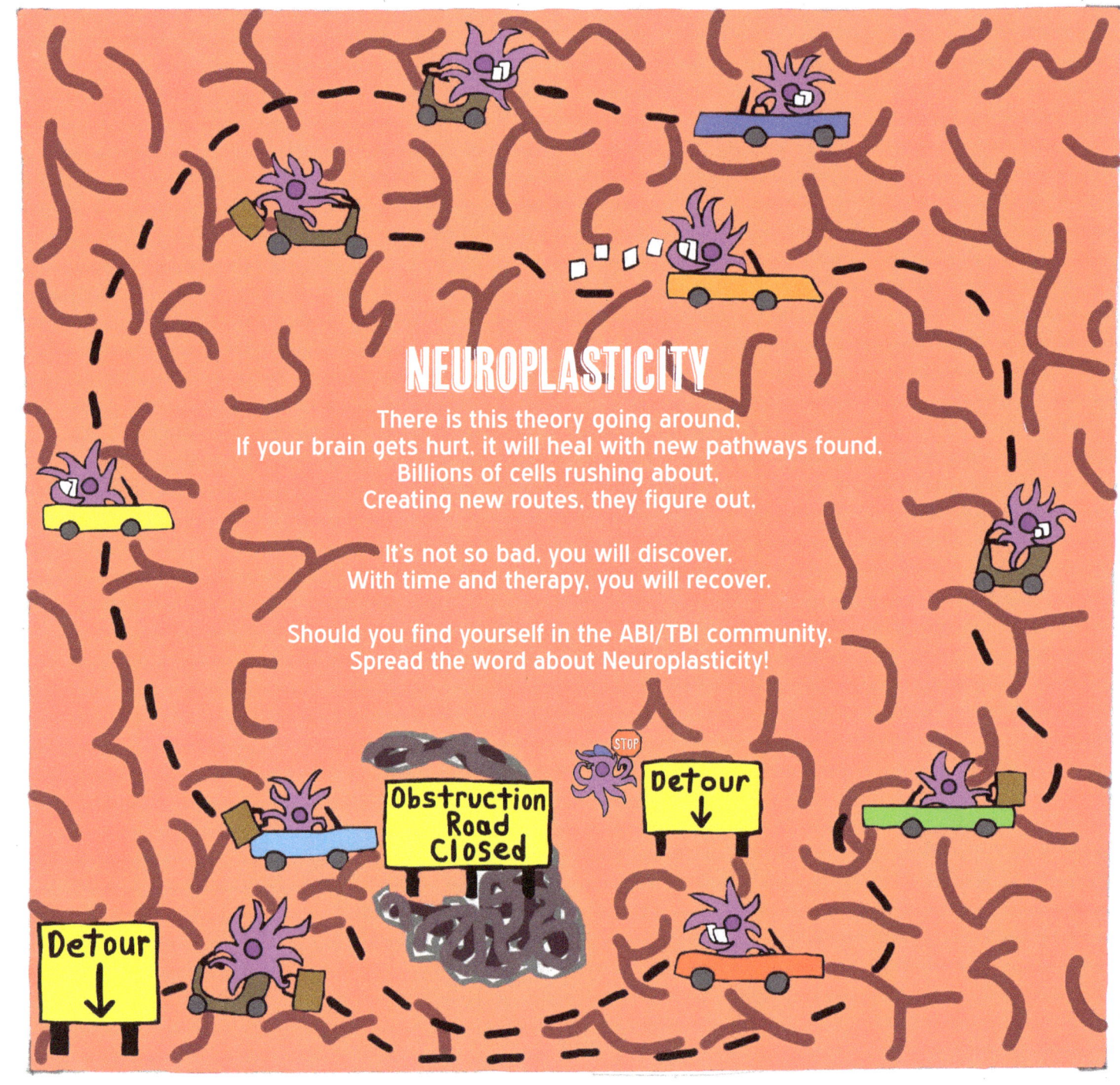

36. VERY BEST OF MEN

During those weak, "why me-woe is me" moments, it is never that difficult to find someone else who is having a tough time of it and fighting their own battles with poor health. Especially those that put on a brave face. My "go-to guy", Mike, was an expat that I met when we first moved over here to North Carolina but when moving back to the UK with his wife, Delia, recently, was diagnosed with muscular dystrophy—a most wretched "muscle wasting" disease. He is a great friend, always the life and soul of any gathering. He has been wheelchair bound for some time now, his six ft. frame hunched over and a little gaunt. Despite everything, he makes every effort to be his usual charming self the moment you arrive on his doorstep. Definitely one of my heroes!

So, to all you "woe is me wusses" out there, look around, find yourself a hero like Mike; sure, a stroke is a major setback, not a death sentence, best you focus on your own battles and move forward; it is not as bad as you think!

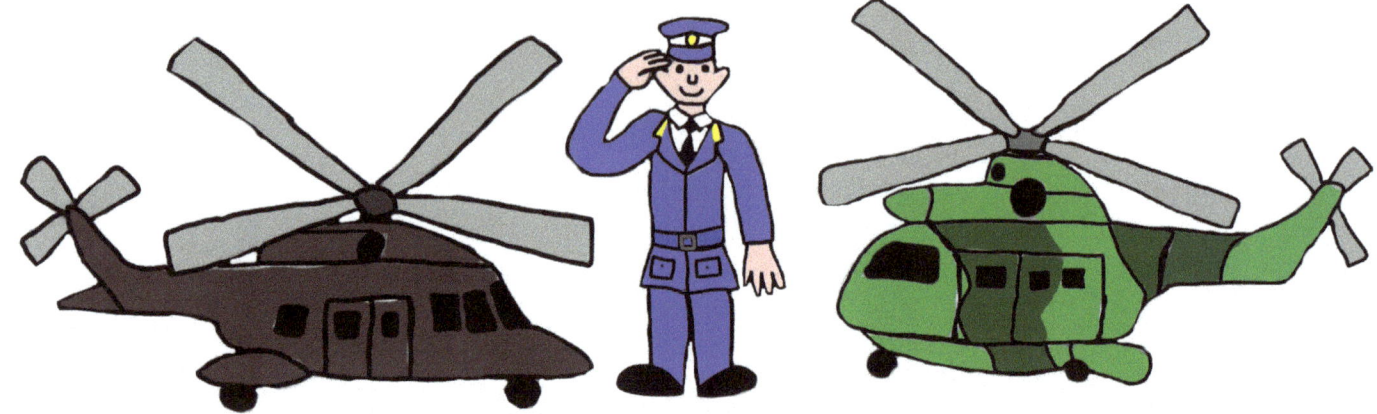

VERY BEST OF MEN

Mike Evans is the best man I met,
A military man, an R-A-F Vet,
A gentle man, with a smile so warm,
Looking so smart in his uniform,

Mike Evans is the best man I've seen,
Barbecue is his preferred cuisine,
Be sure to take care of your waistline,
When Mike serves his infamous loin of swine.

Mike Evans is the best man I know,
He was struck down with MD a few years ago,
To him and all it was a devastating blow,
A worse disease there cannot be,
Where muscles waste so needlessly,
So many reasons for him to feel blue,
Yet, like beacons, his gecko eyes welcomes you.

Mike Evans is the best man forever,
Everyone agrees from me to whomever,
A man truly formidable,
In the whole world there is no better individual.

I can only repeat again and again,
Mike Evans is the very best of men.

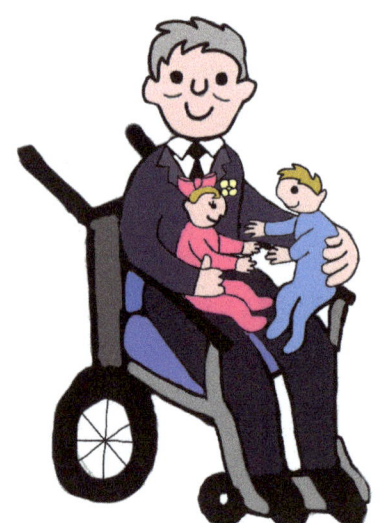

37. ETIQUETTE

[noun]: The Customary code of polite behavior in society or among members of a particular profession or group.

I am proud to say that in England, [many of] my generation was raised to observe and adopt the absolute best etiquette standards from as long as I can remember and of course, starting with those "magic words," please and thank you." But there is so much more; from holding a door open for someone behind you, offering your seat to a lady or an elderly person and so the list went on.

When spending time in any new country it is understandable that there is a potential for cultural differences and possible variations pertaining to overall etiquette and manners. I must say, however, when my family and I moved to North Carolina (nearly) thirty years ago, we were delighted to not only see no diminishment of standard, but it was better in some respects.

Our kids would invite their friends to join us for a family dinner which is the absolute best situation to see how someone was brought up. I cannot count the times I found myself saying, "Please call me Simon, my father was Mr. Barton" and, "thank you, but we can wash the dishes later, please take your seat." As a soccer coach, collectively, our boys always offered to help carry and set up the training equipment before practice then take apart and carry back to my car immediately following. More recently as a stroke survivor, I have been the recipient of countless acts of courtesy and civility.

Now that I have become a fully paid-up member of the less-abled community, I have become an expert on the subject.

So what happens when the same children grow up and learn to drive a car?

Please indulge me my next pet-peeve, which has intensified more so now that I am back behind the wheel of a car and driving myself to various appointments and engagements and consequentially, driving myself (and my wife) crazy!

When I learned to drive back in England, the instructors drummed in the importance of the rear-view mirror and letting others know what your driving objectives were, like using your indicators to "indicate" your intention of making a course change of some kind. In the US, and as usual, they have simplified the English terminology even more so, they call the facility a "Turn Signal", (thus "signaling" to others your intention to turn) and yet, it is seldom used!

The convenience of purchasing fast food through a drive-thru' facility does not entitle you to have a "throw-thru' window" Littering the side of the road is both obnoxious and disrespectful and entitles me to label you a slob.

You can really appreciate how a "deer in headlights" feels when an oncoming driver fails to dip theirs. Just the flick of a switch, how hard is that?

Just as grating as the points above, there is no such thing as a "cruising lane". There is a slow lane and one or two passing/overtaking lanes—if you are not overtaking, then there is every reason to indicate and move over into the slow lane and allow those behind that wish to pass, to overtake in the correct lane(s).

Lastly, what is it about a smart phone that inspires a need to pick it up and look at it and/or text someone? It is bad enough in the middle of a conversation or at the dinner table but in the car, really?

Ultimately, there is absolutely no reason the observance of etiquette should be limited to pedestrians. I do hope that upon reading this reflection, if and when you are in a position to impart advice to someone of the younger generation, you grab their attention; driving would become such a more pleasant and tranquil pastime if we were all a little more respectful and thoughtful. Thank you.

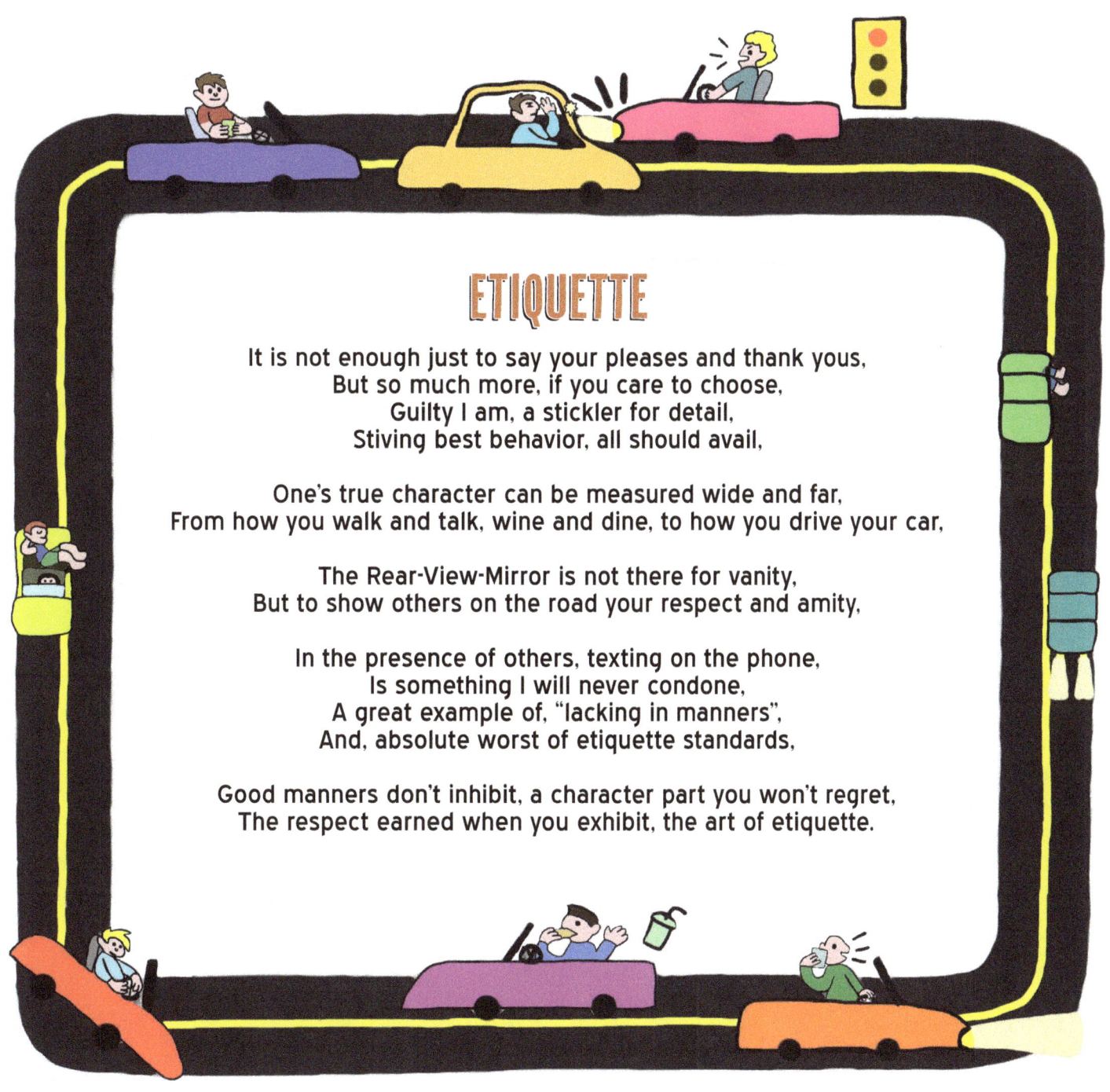

ETIQUETTE

It is not enough just to say your pleases and thank yous,
But so much more, if you care to choose,
Guilty I am, a stickler for detail,
Stiving best behavior, all should avail,

One's true character can be measured wide and far,
From how you walk and talk, wine and dine, to how you drive your car,

The Rear-View-Mirror is not there for vanity,
But to show others on the road your respect and amity,

In the presence of others, texting on the phone,
Is something I will never condone,
A great example of, "lacking in manners",
And, absolute worst of etiquette standards,

Good manners don't inhibit, a character part you won't regret,
The respect earned when you exhibit, the art of etiquette.

38. YOU KNOW YOU'RE OLD

I had my stroke at the age of 52. I left the hospital a few weeks later at the age of 82 and when this book is due to be published, I will have turned 62. These three ages represent how I feel/felt quite aptly during this long journey of mine.

Prior to the stroke, I was quite active and playing a good physical game of tennis most Thursday evenings—I think it fair to say, I was a pretty fit fifty-two-year-old. Upon my release from rehab hospital, I was literally "wheeled" into the car and still in need of 24 hour care from Sarah for two to three weeks following. Despite a slight downturn, mentally with my failure to realize my initial recovery goals, I have since rebounded back and become a pretty fit and spritely 62-year-old with everything to live for. Life is good.

Like many of my generation it is not all plain sailing, I had (and continue) to require assistance for all things "IT", from my iPhone to the Smart TV to my computer, I can sense my children's eyes "rolling" when they see their phone's caller ID—I wonder what he needs help with this time? I can sense them thinking.

I come from two family lines where both grandfathers were quite bald, and the writing was on the cards with my receding hair line in my early 20s, so I knew what was in store. My father and elder brother both needed reading glasses from quite a young age and all these early warning forecasts can be helpful dealing with the psychological effects of getting older, or at least in those areas; but heck, I still figured I had more than enough time to make some good pension money from my business and enjoy many more sets of tennis with a backup sport of golf when younger players were making me huff and puff too much and before I was genuinely too old and unfit to play.

As has been said many times before by accepting and embracing my new self, to a large extent, I have spared the "chips" and I am not concerned with my newly found frailties and limitations and if you wish to hold the door open for me as I limp toward it, or offer me your seat on the bus, I will say, "thank you very much!". "Bring it on," I say.

Anyway, the following set of rhymes are a collection of circumstances I never thought could possibly affect me in these, my middle years, some were already on the horizon, others, however, caught me a little off guard.

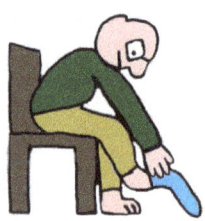 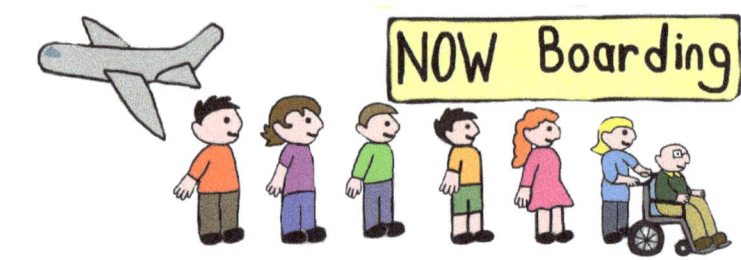

YOU KNOW YOU'RE OLD

When your wife gets there before you to hold open the door,
Your kids have finally realized, you are a total bore,
Putting on your socks has become a major chore, and …
You buy reading glasses in packs of four!

When you never leave home without your walking cane,
You are always first to board the aeroplane, and …
Half the carriage gives up their seats on a one-stop-train!

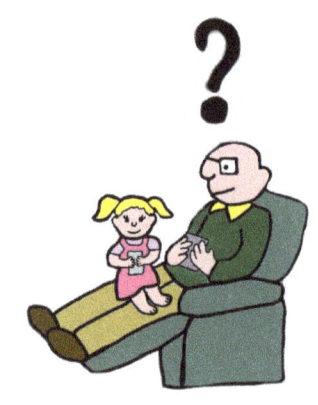

When taking pills seems like a 3-course meal,
You can't see the road for the steering wheel,
Filling your gas is a huge ordeal, and …
.. When praying to God you can't get down to kneel!

When a single-story house becomes your dream home,
You can't remember ever using a comb,
Your grandchild helps you with your iPhone, and …
A day does not pass without you having a moan!

When the day's highlight is the afternoon nap,
A sneeze feels like a heart attack,
Using a golf tee to pick around the teeth you now lack, and …
Farting while walking, helps keep you on track!

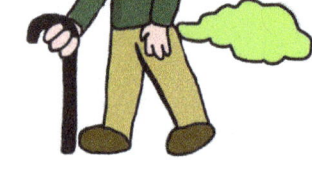 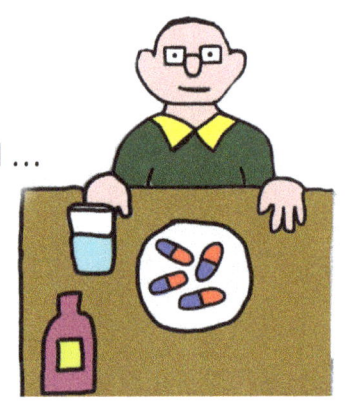

39. MOUSSE ATTACK

As you will have gathered from a couple of my earlier poems, I was not the best behaved child growing up. I was often detained after school for a variety of misdemeanors. Inside the home, I never kept my room tidy, I hated going to bed when I was told so pretended to be asleep under the covers with a flashlight with the latest copy of the Beano comic. I seldom arrived home in time for tea when I was out on my bike with friends. At school, most of my transgressions were limited to scraps in the playground, swearing or maybe answering a teacher back with some kind of derogatory comment and the occasional skiving off—pretty minor stuff mostly. However, I did manage to graduate high school well enough to get into a small engineering college which I also graduated! I think they called kids like me, "late bloomers".

In my new role as a grandfather, and a benefit of the stroke, I now have a little more time to help contribute and mold our grandchildren. In this respect, recently, I was in the process of giving my granddaughter a lecture about the importance of behaving well, my wife turned and looked at me with eyes that said, "yeah right, you can talk." Which reminded me of the following event (that still haunts me to this day).

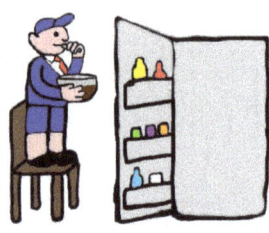

MOUSSE ATTACK

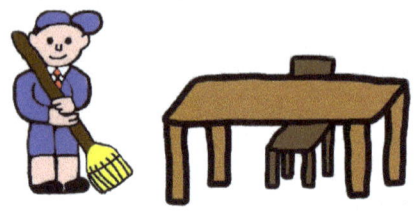

Questionably behaved when I was a lad,
Always in trouble for being bad,
Often my sister said, "I'm telling Dad!"

I don't know why I came to be mean,
I must have gained someone else's gene,
Punishments seemed like a daily routine,

So, I got home from school one afternoon,
Aching from hunger, I had to eat soon,
Without hesitation, I went to the fridge,
There had to something in there,
I could binge,

And there it was! A bowl crystal-gleaming,
Caught my eye with that
"lip-smacking" feeling,
I was not very tall, so grabbed me a chair,
With tiptoes and fingertips, it got me there,

Inside the bowl all creamy and velvet,
A substance so dreamy, I just had to get it!

I didn't need much, just a taste of the stuff,
Two, three maybe four spoons,
should be enough,
It slipped down my throat, all chocolatey-cool,
I was appetized and satisfied in no time at all,

Made sure the kitchen was as
clean as I found it,
Using the broom, I swept all around it,
I had to be careful not to leave any trace,
I washed my hands and cleaned up my face,
Quite meticulous with the time that I spent,
Don't be frivolous, be sublime, act innocent!

The front door slams,
"oh-no, she's come home!
I've got homework, I'm staying in my room,
Five minutes later when she
discovers the ruse,
Loud came the scream,
"WHO ATTACKED MY MOUSSE!?"

Us kids were all summoned
and to stand in a line,
She was looking for clues, just one guilty sign,

"It wasn't me," in turn, we all said,
The culprit was clear when
my face turned red,

"Three hours I spent making this dessert!
"... For our good friends tonight -
Bessie and Bert,"
With so little time, ingredients I've squat,
If I had a gun, I would have you shot!
Your sentence now... is to eat the whole lot!"

One hour later and fat as can be,
I finished the bowl quite diligently,
When Mother succumbed and showed
sympathy,

The lesson was harsh, almost child abuse,
And since that day, never again
did I ever have mousse!

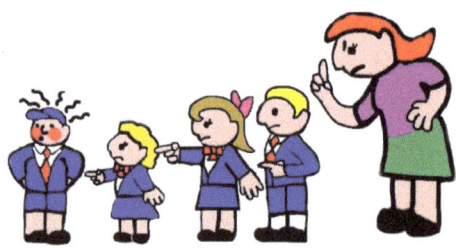

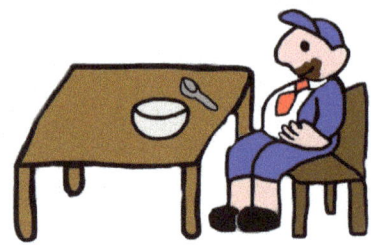

BAD RHYMES, NO REASON

40. BIG MR. MUFFET

Pre stroke, my ideal weekend day would be a North Carolina spring/early summer day (sunny, low humidity but not exceeding 85 deg. F/ 30 deg. C) and would have me getting up as the sun rises, spending an hour or two clearing a couple of chores before heading off for a nice early tee-time at a local golf course with a couple of my best mates followed by a beer or two afterward in the clubhouse. Returning home quite happy with my game along with the social banter. Upon arrival, I immediately head for the bathtub for a 20–30-minute soak and rejuvenation in a hot, (herbally salted) bath. The whole day, however, could be ruined when reaching said bathtub, I find a large, hairy spider sitting there!

I used to think I was a reasonably tough/macho sort of guy, but when it comes to spiders, I am the ultimate "wimpy-wuss", I must confess.

Poststroke the issue is not as relevant, first, because I am unable to grip a golf club with both hands, so I don't play at all and second, I don't take baths anymore—I tried a couple of years ago but found that whilst it was relatively easy getting in, it was quite a different matter getting out!!

It so happened that to save space (when it was not needed), Sarah kept our grandson's potty in the guest bathroom's bathtub which is seldom used. And when the little lad says "I wanna go poo-poo!" you jolly well better stop what you are doing and go fetch the potty, tout suite! On one occasion, the alarm was raised, and even at "the speed of Simon", I got there in time. As soon as I lifted the thing, this vicious, ugly 8 legged monster got down on its haunches looking like it was about to propel itself up onto my shoulder to bite and take chunks out of my neck! My old fear was still there. After delivering the potty, I told Sarah, that there was a seriously dangerous creature that could compromise the grandkids safety and required her immediate attention, but I needed to go straight to my office and write something down for my new book—being the wimpy-wuss, I (still) was!

It's a shame that when having a stroke we don't get to choose the bits of our previous selves we want to keep in exchange for those areas we could benefit from losing!

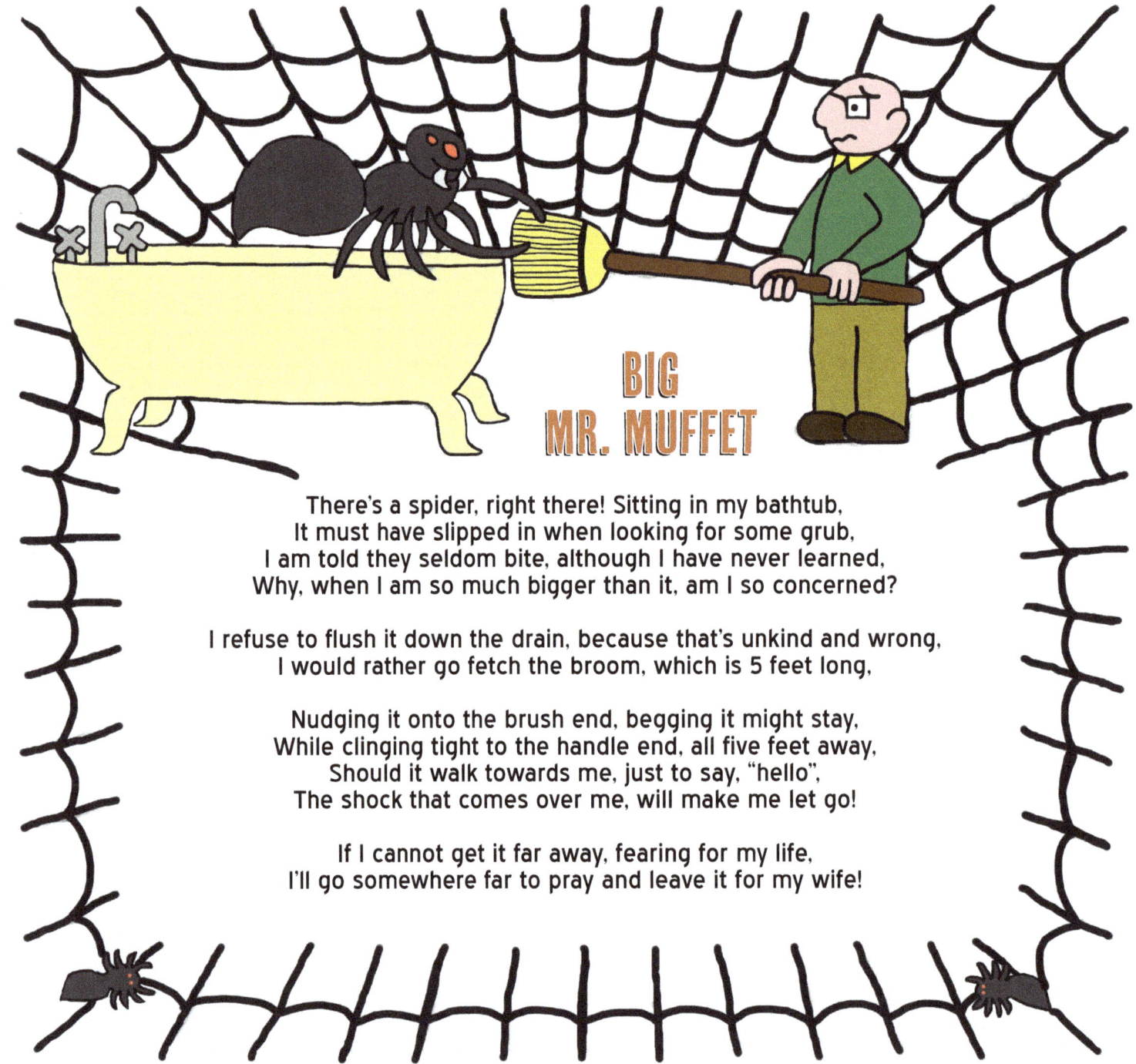

BIG MR. MUFFET

There's a spider, right there! Sitting in my bathtub,
It must have slipped in when looking for some grub,
I am told they seldom bite, although I have never learned,
Why, when I am so much bigger than it, am I so concerned?

I refuse to flush it down the drain, because that's unkind and wrong,
I would rather go fetch the broom, which is 5 feet long,

Nudging it onto the brush end, begging it might stay,
While clinging tight to the handle end, all five feet away,
Should it walk towards me, just to say, "hello",
The shock that comes over me, will make me let go!

If I cannot get it far away, fearing for my life,
I'll go somewhere far to pray and leave it for my wife!

BAD RHYMES, NO REASON

41. BREAK A LEG

At around 18 years of age, I was invited to audition (and subsequently offered) my first proper acting role for a local amateur theatrical society, albeit a relatively small part, I was to play the brother of the central character, Ronnie Winslow, in the play titled The Winslow Boy, by Sir Terrance Rattigan. Ironically, in the story, Ronnie Winslow was expelled from his school when he was suspected of stealing—I could have played that part without reading the script!!

Actually, I enjoyed the experience, especially considering the few positive critiques I earned following the production (mainly from members of my own family that came to see it) but it was enjoyable enough to stay on within the group and participate in a few other productions (Christmas Pantomimes and a couple of one act competitions we entered).

Without doubt, the process of dealing with one's lack of self-confidence and overall nervousness was more than compensated by the feeling of satisfaction having achieved the feat reasonably successfully. Further, this background of acting in public would greatly assist my career as a public speaker in the areas of manufacturing engineering I would move into in later years.

The expression, "Break a Leg" is usually offered to someone that is about to undertake some kind of performance in front of an audience (and particularly an actor about to go on stage), ultimately, it is a gesture of good luck. There are many theories about the true origin for the term. the one that I tend to favor is based on first, that most theater personnel are notoriously superstitious and pessimistic to the extent that they believed in opposite and negative consequences following remarks of good intention (saying "good luck" could become the "kiss of death", etc.) so they were always on the lookout for an alternative type of positive gesture. It so happens that during the eighteenth and nineteenth centuries, actors were only paid for the time they were on stage, i.e. on the stage side of the "legs" (tall narrow curtains to the side of the stage that are designed to obscure the view of the audience) The only people permitted around these leg areas were actors waiting to enter the stage; stagehands, and maybe an understudy or the production's prompt etc. So, hoping you "break a leg" in this case, is hoping you get on stage, with success and good fortune to follow … and voila, "break a leg!

I guess, between my late teens until my marriage I appeared in a production of some kind at least twenty times and within my engineering career, I spoke publicly on many more occasions. I can honestly say there was not a single event, regardless of size or significance, that I did not feel awful and fearful of failure and this sensation was at its peak 6-12 hours before showtime and would grow to the point of almost wanting to throw up just 5 minutes before going on which I came to learn was largely influenced by the level and extent of care and preparation I (and my companions) had undertaken beforehand.

Returning to the workplace within a few months of being released from hospital thinking that I was capable of resuming the type(s) of work I was doing pre stroke was a big mistake. Looking back at all the typos I was making in simple email communications combined with my inability to chair internal staff meetings and maintain some level of composure, control and focus should have served as a clue to my limitations but despite the (sometimes strong) suggestions from others close to me at the time, I remained oblivious and in total denial of these shortfalls.

It so happened that I was booked to present a technical lecture at McCormick Convention Center in Chicago later that year where the subject matter related to a new (patented) technology we had developed. My VP of Engineering at the time, Michael Gaunce, said he would be happy to do the lecture in my place, but again, I was too stubborn to listen and said that I was quite capable. I might be apprehensive because of my apparent loss of confidence but "it will be alright on the night" and I would rise to the challenge, after all, it was still a few months away—loads of time. Of course, he was totally right with hindsight because I failed miserably! As late as the previous evening I was still struggling to put my PowerPoint slides together and went to bed tired and depressed and very concerned. I barely slept a wink that night. Fortunately, Mike was available on the day because he was supporting our booth at the accompanying exhibition and at least I had the good sense to ask him to stand by—just in case he was needed to contribute. As it happened, after the conference chair introduced me, I got up to speak, opened my mouth took an embarrassing pause and just broke into tears—right in front of everyone! For some reason, I received some applause as I was accompanied off the stage like a "wobbling jelly". Without hesitation, Mike stepped in and provided a flawless presentation on our behalf. Phew!

Following that terrible experience, I concluded that my public speaking days were over. That was until I met Dr. Jamila Minga at North Carolina Central University who, at the time, was researching language and communication disorders associated with right hemisphere brain injuries and somehow, she encouraged me to try again and provide a talk to some of her SLP students about my recovery experiences to date—probably one of the best things that has happened since the stroke.

The fear and dread I have felt prior to speaking publicly is not unique; some people refuse to do it at all and I remember the great, late Shakespearean actor, Sir Lawrence Olivier once saying that the level of nauseousness he felt prior to going on would often serve as an indicator to the quality of the performance he was about to deliver; "these feelings of insecurity are quite natural and should be embraced", he said.

Since the talk at NCCU and the publication of my first book, I have had the good fortune to speak at a number of other engagements, some as small as ten to twenty in a conference room type setting and others that might involve up to two to three hundred in an auditorium or theater environment. The sensations I feel before going on remain the same but on balance, I think most of the experiences have been worthwhile and quite therapeutic and beneficial—particularly with regard to bolstering one's self-esteem—a personality trait that is often lost to stroke survivors.

I fear that I am still a little monotone with my public speaking delivery, but it is the one area of my journey that I can check off as being almost as good as I once was. Yay!

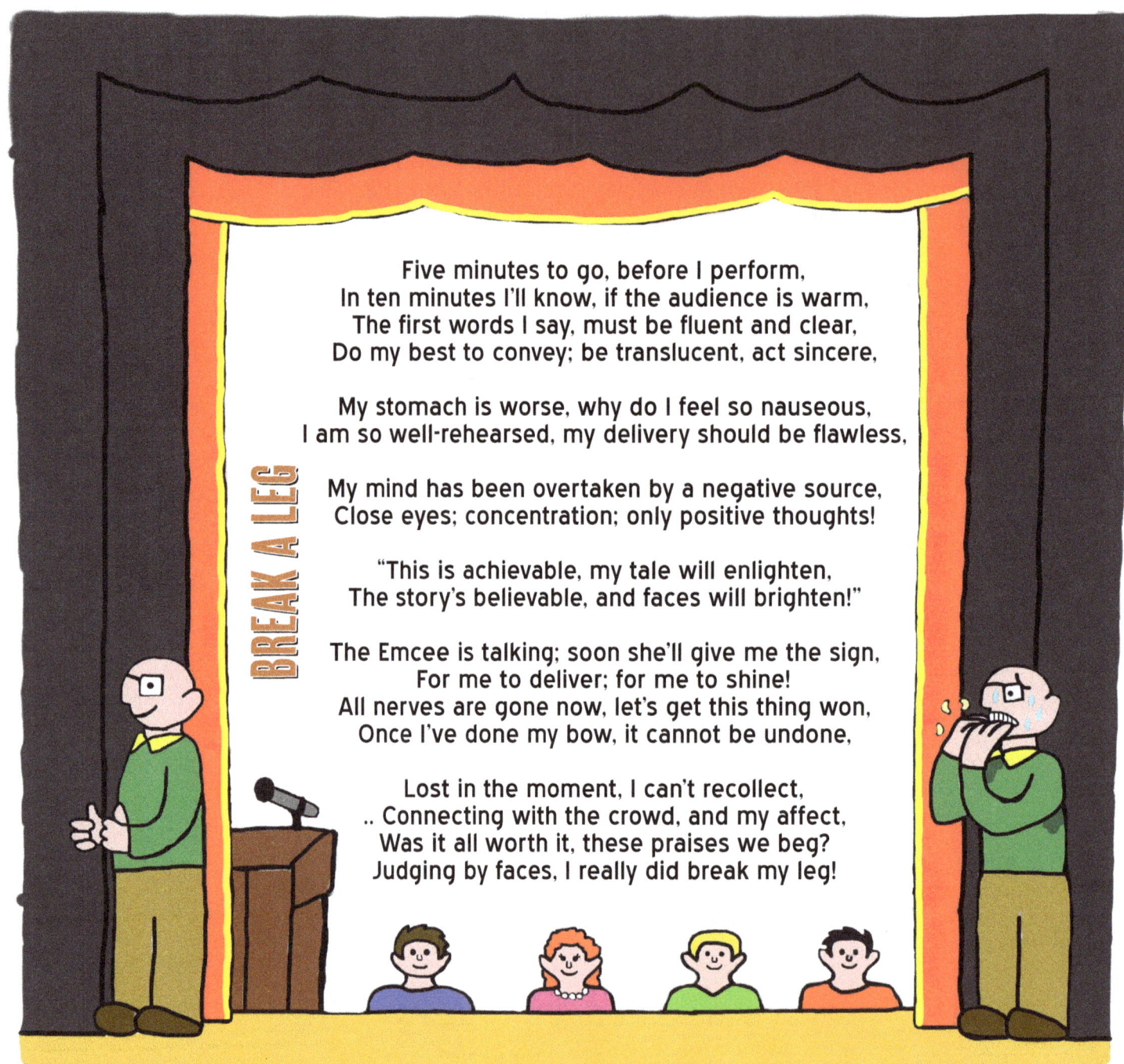

42. SIXTEEN

As a boy, I used to regard golf as an "old man's sport". I took one lesson in England during my college days with a couple of classmates and this introduction to the game of golf was just enough for me not to embarrass myself and feel reasonably confident enough to accept the occasional invitation to play with my dad, should he be so inclined to extend the offer. My interest grew to the extent that before our kids were born, Sarah was happy for me to sneak in a Saturday round two to three times a month. I was not very good, but I could hit the ball so that it would go up in the air (most times) and to a reasonable distance although I must confess, I spent more time looking for the ball than I did hitting the thing! With the arrival of our children, weekends became too precious to spend half a day away, at least until a job offer came my way to work in America and everything changed.

Culturally, golf was a completely different pastime to the UK's way of playing the sport. In England, indifferent weather meant less opportunity to play; the process of simply drawing back the curtains first thing in the morning would have me saying, "oh dear, I don't feel like playing today, I will call the guys and let them know." Secondly, golf courses were more sporadic which meant joining a club quite far away, a club that would have rules, dress codes, snobby members, and overall higher costs.

So, we arrive in America, and from the first day in the office, the most common question seemed to be, "you do play golf, right?" Everyone played; it was the place to get to know you; it was the place we discussed business; it was the place we told our best jokes. Playing golf was the opportunity to escape from the office, our family, problems, and life in general; the golf course was simply the best place to escape, period! Inside a twenty-minute drive from the office there were at least fifteen golf courses to choose from, all good quality and affordable. And, neither of them had a "more than my jobs worth" "official" coming up to you to say, "your shorts need to be longer to cover the knee-caps! And your shirt must have a collar" etc. In addition, in North Carolina, most favor the use of a golf cart (the expression "fat and happy" comes to mind), also most observe and practice a "ready golf" (speed of play) philosophy, which ultimately means that we can play eighteen holes within a couple of hours comfortably. Straight after work, we could get in nine holes plus a beer in the clubhouse afterward and still be home for supper with a sympathetic spouse, "yeah, it was a really tough day today, dear, the phone wouldn't stop ringing—couldn't get a break all day! Please pass the mustard, thank you."

The one disadvantage of playing golf in my newly adopted country is that most of the Americans I played with were jolly good players! The standard that got me by in England was nowhere near close enough to feel comfortable on a Pinehurst level/type golf course with three Americans making up the foursome. I needed to improve; I needed to practice and play more; I needed to get myself shooting below the one hundred mark for eighteen holes consistently which would equate to a golf handicap of just under thirty. Which is good, right? Certainly better but sadly, still not good enough! My father, who purchased a vacation home in North Carolina so he and Mother could get closer to their grandchildren a couple of times a year; even at the ripe old age of seventy-five was playing golf consistently to a fifteen (or better) handicap. Inevitably meaning that I had to practice and play more. I had to get better, and so this game, that I had very little appreciation for initially, was now taking over my life. I even joined a local golf club and every time I played, I would faithfully enter my score onto the club's computer where it would calculate and churn out my latest, amended handicap, and gradually, I was becoming my father! Truly evidenced when returning home, by the manner, in which the front door closed or slammed thus indicating the quality of the morning's play and whether it was better that the kids kept their distance. With each following year, the handicap had to be lowered further and I needed to practice and play more!

Eventually, the time came when I started to play golf quite well and consistently posted a score in the low to mid-eighties and I remember very well the day and the feeling of elation when the club's computer said my handicap went down from 17.2 to 16.4!

Sadly, the hemiplegia I gained resulting from my stroke means that I am unable to grip anything with my left hand, and for a right-handed golfer, the left hand (the leading hand) is most important.

I did try to play a couple of times, one-handed, but considering the level I had attained, I soon lost my enthusiasm. But following the principle of acceptance, I have learned to be happy and reserve my interest now to the occasional TV event and just a couple of personal memories. Not the end of the world.

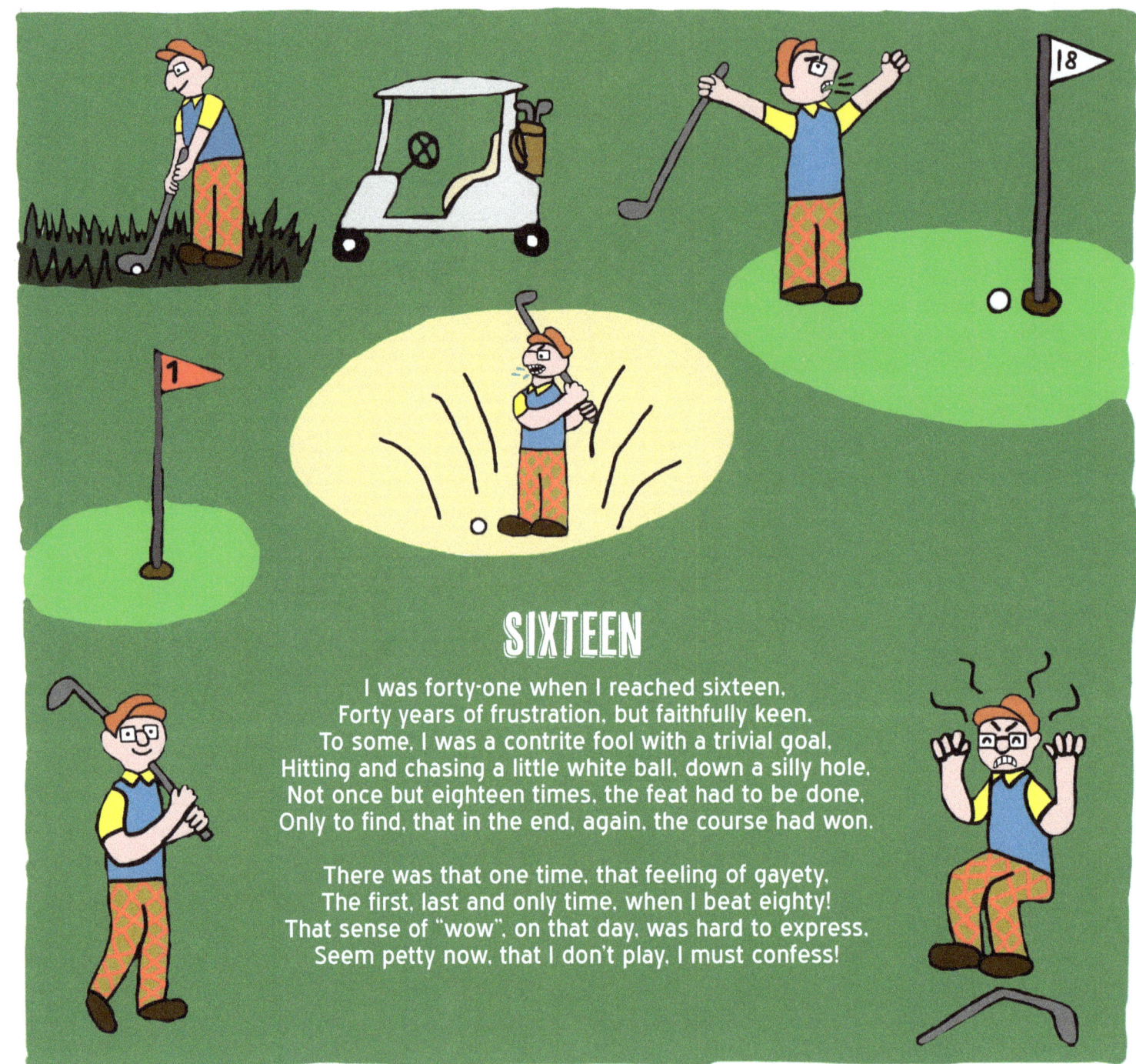

SIXTEEN

I was forty-one when I reached sixteen,
Forty years of frustration, but faithfully keen.
To some, I was a contrite fool with a trivial goal,
Hitting and chasing a little white ball, down a silly hole.
Not once but eighteen times, the feat had to be done,
Only to find, that in the end, again, the course had won.

There was that one time, that feeling of gayety,
The first, last and only time, when I beat eighty!
That sense of "wow", on that day, was hard to express.
Seem petty now, that I don't play, I must confess!

43. NO NEWS TODAY

As your average family man and senior manager, I failed to keep up with the news. Before the stroke, I was seldom later than 7.00 a.m. in the office and rarely earlier than 7.00 p.m. before arriving home each evening. My exposure to the TV news was limited to the weekends and/or when there was something particularly newsworthy that caught my interest. Hurricane Katrina was such an event I remember, for example.

Poststroke, my daily routine has me eating my yoghurt breakfast after my walk (in front of TV News) and I might take a nap later in the afternoon intending to drop off when watching one of the news channels.

Despite so called "journalistic objectivity", over the past few years, I have found it extremely difficult to find a news outlet that is truly unbiased and concerned only with reporting the news as purely factual information. I think it a sad reflection of today's society as a whole that the media moguls think that the only way they can increase circulation and ratings, is through some kind of cocktail of innuendo and opinion—supposedly because as a public, no longer are we capable of digesting and interpreting said news in a simple and impartial manner.

It has become so bad that I think there should be a movement to have the word "news" excluded from all media outlets that abuse the word unless they have earned the privilege to incorporate it. I am dead set against any censoring of free speech—accordingly, during the interim period as they try to get their act together, they can simply replace the word, "news" with "views". So, from now on, it will be "Fox Views" on the one side with the counter channel, "Cable Views Network", on the other. Paper media like the New York Post and Washington Post will now sell "ViewsPapers"

I volunteer myself to take on the important role and position of the "adjudicator" with full authority to identify and award the word "news" (with appropriate commensurate salary and benefits, of course) for those organizations that wish to apply for the acknowledgement. Please propose this idea to your member of congress, and at the same time, don't forget to vote for me! Thank you. I think it a position that even a dimwit with half a brain, like me, can take on and undertake as well as the next person.

This need to take a side or a rigid viewpoint is not limited to politics, sadly. Over the past few years, I have witnessed the line drawing that goes on between conventional and modern medical practices. Every Tuesday, I undertake a fairly rigorous "workout" with a local and talented Chiropractor, Dr. Graham Clements of Chiropractic Partners of Raleigh. With the absence of conventional physical & occupational therapies, he has taken on the mantle of working my hemiplegic left side. Of course, as a chiropractor, he is a "Quack", or at least as far as many on the "traditional" side of healthcare, are concerned. Many insurance companies do not recognize and cover reasonable treatment plans. All I know, is that I feel stronger and better every day resulting from his weekly intervention. Perish the thought, should he have the audacity to prescribe or recommend some kind of medical cannabis—the height of quackery!!

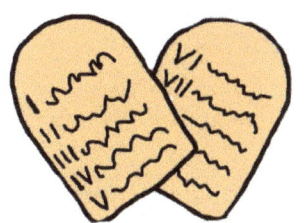 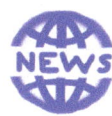 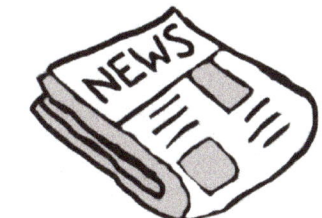

NO NEWS TODAY

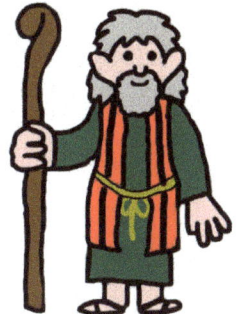

As a boy, I thought TV was great,
Until Dad came home and changed it to "News at Eight,"
A boring man wearing a tie and suit,
How this was fun, I couldn't compute,
I had no interest in anything he said,
Signaling to me. It was time for bed,

As I got older, with kids of my own,
On went the News, when I got home,
The Anchor was still dull as he delivered the news,
It was interesting to me but made my kids snooze.

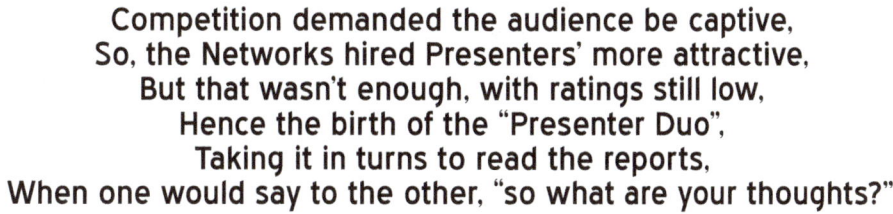

Competition demanded the audience be captive,
So, the Networks hired Presenters' more attractive,
But that wasn't enough, with ratings still low,
Hence the birth of the "Presenter Duo",
Taking it in turns to read the reports,
When one would say to the other, "so what are your thoughts?"

Instead of the news being boring but true,
It's become inuendo and a biased view,
Watching the news now, makes me feel blue.

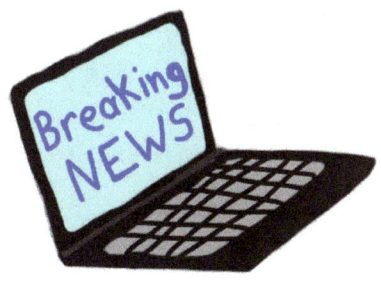 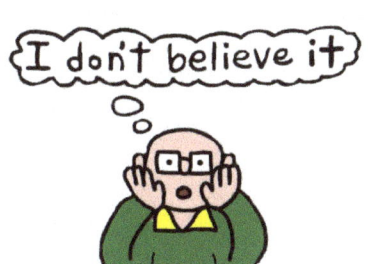 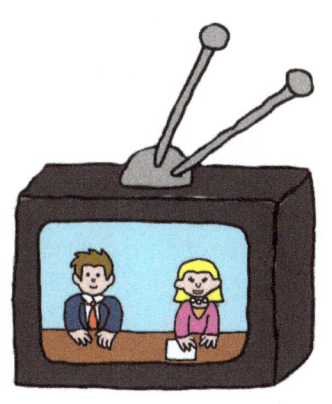

Reflections, Ramblings & Rantings of a Rancorous Stroke Survivor

44. ETHEL AND THE BRIGHT LIME GREEN TRAILER

According to the Centers for Disease Control and Prevention (CDC), "Stroke is the leading cause of serious long-term disability. Further, every year, around 800,000 people in the United States have a stroke and about 600,000 of these are first or new strokes." They go on to state that stroke related costs associated with healthcare and time off work, in the United States, came to nearly $53 Billion between the years 2017 and 2018.

In short, it can be very expensive to recuperate from a stroke event.

In the second chapter, I suggested that I believed my stroke was deserved because it was self-inflicted primarily due to my work and social lifestyle at the time. Combined with my poststroke experiences to date, this uphill and almost insurmountable battle had Ms. Lynn Caulberg, Chiropractic assistant to Dr. Graham Clements reminding me to recount the story I told her about a particular time in my early family life which was also not only self-inflicted, prolonged (with high and low points), but also cost more money than we had.

When the kids were still less than seven years old, we moved to a smallholding in the rural county of Derbyshire England, the property boasted around 2 ½ acres of land with a couple of outbuildings for farm animals. At the time. It seemed like a good idea to expose our children to some "country life". Despite the fact that we had not equated the cost and time associated with fence repairs and overall property upkeep, there were some stables which with some good, adjacent grazing pastures, allowed us to offer a young local girl, Katy, a place to keep and ride her pony for the welcome return of free babysitting services. But it didn't stop there …

In addition to a small stable block, there was a fenced pen area and a chicken coop, so we had to get ourselves some chickens with the hope of some fresh eggs for breakfast. I don't remember who it was but, "have you ever had a goose egg for breakfast?" said one of us to the others, and so we welcomed Bessie and Tessie to the yard. I remember our visiting three-year-old nephew one weekend, getting attacked by these birds that were twice his size. He told us only recently (now in his 30s) that he still has nightmares from the ordeal. Geese are the most pernicious, aggressive, poop-generating, machines—nobody in their right mind should keep! But it got worse ...

There was also a pigsty on the property and Sarah had always loved pigs. Typically Simon, I had to buy her the sweetest little piglet for an anniversary present one time. It turned out that Doris, as she was called, was from the "Large White" breed, she didn't stay sweet and little for very long. When we left for America around seven years later, Doris weighed around 5,000 pounds.

At no time did we ever properly consider the overall cost of such a lifestyle. The food for Doris alone was greater than all the humans combined living in the house. But then it got worse.

It so happened that Sarah at around the age of 12 had riding lessons and enjoyed the experience and heck, we had a spare stable. We just had to get ourselves a horse! We were at least sensible enough to know that we could not afford some kind of thoroughbred. So, we scoured the local papers until a horse became available that we could financially justify. Eventually, we found one, an elderly mare, around 16 hands (about 64 inches from front hoof to shoulder). She was quite large and almost as wide as she was tall, and since that statistic reminded us of my Great Aunt (not long passed), we named her, "Ethel".

But what is the point of having a horse if you are not going to ride her? We needed a saddle and tackle and Sarah had to be safe and look the part. Add in the mix of horse-riding attire and a helmet, Ethel was not the best financial investment I ever made. But it got worse ...

What is the point of riding a horse on your own? With nobody to compare to and very few horsey type people one can associate with. We just had to show her, we had to compete at some local events. We had to get ourselves a horse trailer!

Having never bought a horse trailer before, I was shocked to see how expensive they were. The more streamlined looking and lighter they were, the more money they cost. It follows, therefore, that the trailer we ended up buying was not a state-of-the-art, streamlined looking aluminum type, rather it was an ugly looking box that had a welded steel chassis frame under a heavy wood paneled body, it was over twenty years old and quite dilapidated. At the time, I had a 1.8L, front-wheel drive family estate car (station wagon) not the sort of vehicle designed to tow heavy loads. After having the necessary towbar conversion, we went to pick up the trailer. Even with nothing in it, the effort just to move forward had me selecting a lower gear until there were no more lower gears to select from. The poor car was screaming and practically overheating getting to a respectable 30 mph. Somehow, we made it home and found a nice space to tuck it away and spend a couple of days giving it a bright, lime-green paint job that would help to use up some of those many gallons we purchased during a weak moment when a local business was selling it in bulk (and very cheap), one day. But then it got worse …

Derbyshire is regarded as one of the most beautiful counties in England. Jane Austen's book, Pride and Prejudice has the primary house, "Pemberley", situated in Derbyshire. Derbyshire is not renowned for its beauty because it is flat. No, Derbyshire is famed for its rolling, heather covered hills. Big hills! Hills that a car filled with a family like mine towing a horse trailer like ours, carrying a horse like Ethel has to climb! But even the effort of getting to the various venues are not the worse part …

In England, your average, local, horse gymkhana, is never held in an enclosed building with a nice tarmac covered car park. It is usually situated on a remote farmer's field in the middle of nowhere. In England, it rains a lot, and a field will get wet and muddy. Most times. the field had cattle grazing in it right up to the day before. We arrive and driving slowly, we start looking for a parking space—preferably away from the "hoity-toity-lord-of-the-manor" type people. People identifiable by their gleaming four-wheel drive Land Rover-Range Rovers coupled to their streamlined looking, aluminum, lightweight trailers. No, we have no interest in hearing about the private school "Priscilla" attends or the thoroughbred horse she got for her birthday. No, we are going to park further away, down the hill a bit …

A few hours later, there we are, dusk beginning to fall, all packed up and ready to go. Trailer hitched to the car and Ethel contently secured in place. It had been a nice day; the rain was lighter than forecast, the kids got to have some ice cream and see their mother place fourth in one of the (over 25) cross country events. I point us up the slope, put my foot down and see brown spray flying past my side window. With wheels spinning it was patently clear we were not going anywhere! Before I can get out the car to place some straw under the wheels, a young lady trots up on a very fine looking horse and as I wind my window down, says, "How do you do? My name is Priscilla Parker-Barnes, I see you are having some trouble, let me get my father to tow you out, he has a four-wheel drive Land Rover-Range Rover you know, I will tell him where you are and to look out for the car pulling a bright, lime-green trailer." And off she went. Around 15 minutes later, Mr. Parker ("IV", I think he said) arrived and as it would turn out he was not only quite amenable but got us back to the road quite effortlessly.

Since the stroke, the embarrassment I feel on those occasions when I break into tears in a public setting pales in comparison when remembering the time when, as we drive home, climbing a hill with Ethel in tow, foot hard down on the floor accelerator and the kids in the back are shouting in unison, "faster Dad, you have to go faster!" And as I look in my side mirror, I watch open-mouthed as a cyclist overtakes me.

ETHEL AND THE LIME GREEN TRAILER

Ethel, the mare, had a very large backside,
Beyond compare, her weight was quite immense,
The trailer to move her was twice as wide
Towing them both proved adverse and little sense.

But tow her, we did—gyrating many hill and dale,
Motor exceeded—vibrating the wheel, that really shook me,
Just when I thought my car would fail,
A cyclist overtook me!

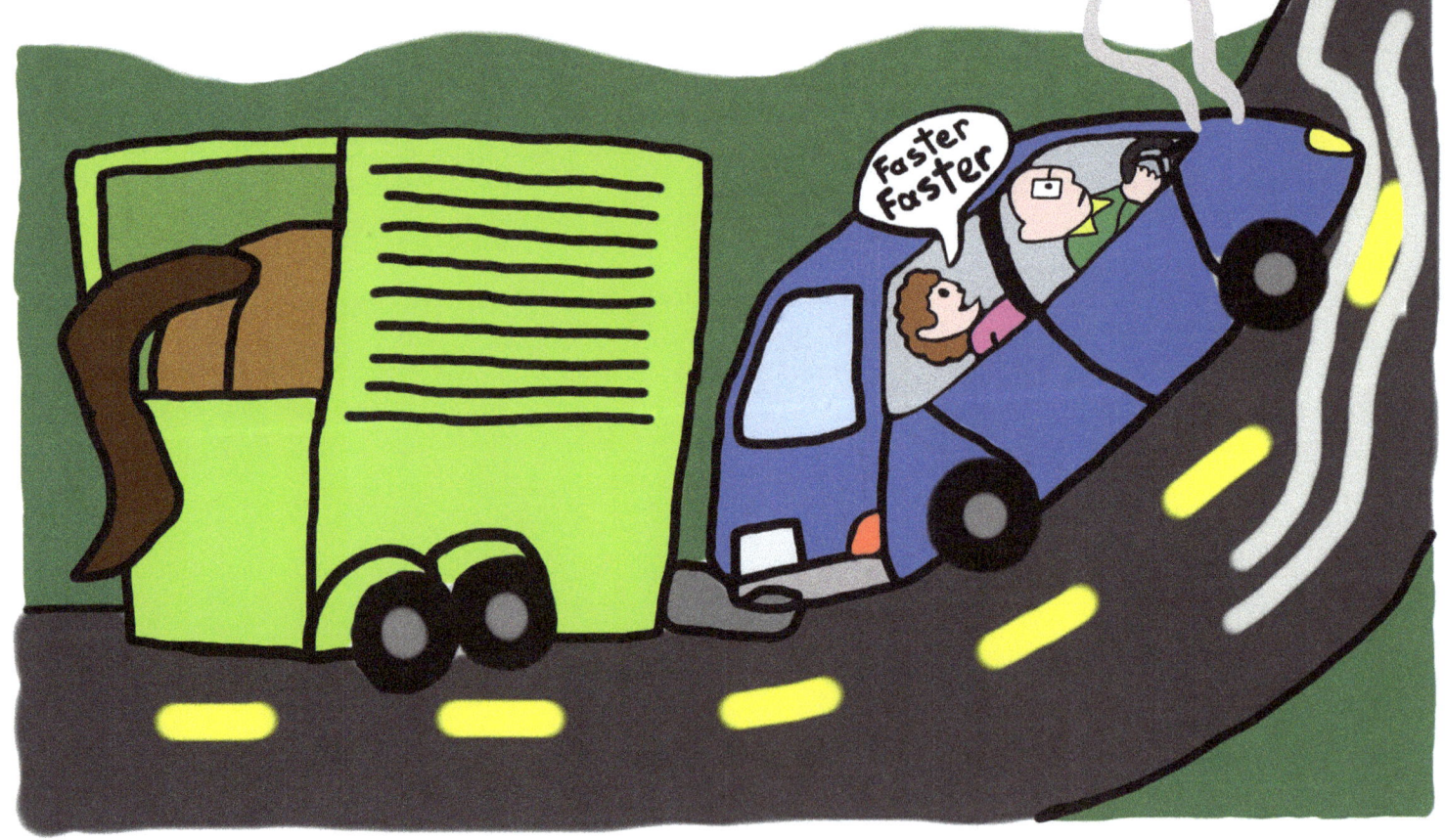

45. FREEDOM (QUEST FOR INDEPENDENCE)

When I was undergoing one of my initial physical therapy treatments in the rehab hospital, I remember being interrupted by a stroke survivor, Shawn Fleck, that received treatment from the same PT a few months earlier, and upon seeing Shawn, the PT commented, "Hi Shawn, how come you are looking so happy?" Shawn, with a huge grin on his face, replied, "I had to come and tell you … I passed my driving test yesterday!". At the time, I could not understand his euphoria (big deal, I thought).

Little did I know then that I would undergo the exact same feeling of elation when I passed my driving exam many months later. The moment I was admitted to hospital I was placed under 24 hour care from the doctors and nurses—even my bed was alarmed to signal the nursing station any attempt I made to get up. When I felt I needed to go to the toilet, I would spend ages trying to beat that pesky alarm rather than press the buzzer for a nurse to bring me a bedpan. It became the contest I never won. The best result I ever achieved was getting one leg out from under the covers, all the way to the knee! But as I slowly pushed for those extra few inches, that grating, high pitched noise broke the silence, shortly followed with a very vexed nurse poking her head through the doorway, with dagger eyes and shrieking voice, "Mr. Barton, you were not trying to get out of bed, were you?" "No, not me, ma'am" I would reply, "I think I was just tossing and turning when it went off—it woke me up, it did; I was having a really nice dream at the time. I think you should disable it; I think it is too sensitive" I would argue, but she (rightly) saw through me, ignored my lame defense and went about her business.

The typical daily routine at the hospital would involve a bed bath each morning followed by a light breakfast and then hoisted by a (Hoyer) crane lift from the bed into a wheelchair and taken to various therapies or the cafeteria at lunch and supper times but always returning to my "cell" of a bed in between times.

It was a great relief to be told I was eventually allowed to go home only to find my wife would take on the role of "mother of mothers". She was given a crash course in all the dos and don'ts as far as making sure I did not "come a cropper" through some self-inflicted act of stupidity. She washed me, dressed me, fed me, and then ferried me to my various medical appointments—sat in on all of them and then reminded me most of the rotten bits all the way home.

I have often thought that the immediate consequence of surviving a stroke is like going back to when we were a young child; we have to learn how to walk, talk, and fend for ourselves all over again. The major difference now being that we have some recollection of knowing how it was done prior to the stroke event but now being told that we "can't" or that we had "to do it together" or simply, "just do it better," only added to the resentment. It is understandable why many marriages become strained to the point of breaking down. Each partner finds themselves in the unfamiliar territory of either being the patient or the caregiver. I cannot speak for my wife—I really do not know how she put up with me; I was a needy, lousy, demanding, miserable, and most ungrateful patient and S.O.B of a husband much of the time, those first couple of years.

The quest for independence was always there but came on so gradually, I barely realized its significance. The first of the clues came when Katie Stephens PT, NCS, had me upright, away from my wheelchair and walking for the first time. Tears rolled down my cheeks as I shuffled across her clinic floor as visible indication that good things can happen, even to the worst of us— even to me.

The fact is that only with hindsight, many years later, did I realize that from that first encounter with Shawn, I knew nothing about anything; at that time, I was just a puppet totally dependent on the hands of its Marionettes. Despite being told, I could not possibly envisage what this post stroke journey would entail—my journey had not even begun.

Other milestones came along. Sarah let me get myself out of bed when she thought I was capable, walk to the bathroom, shower myself, brush my teeth, and with a newly fitted banister rail, I could even get down the stairs on my own and make us both a cup of tea—I struggled getting back up the stairs because the handrail was now on the wrong side, my weak side. But with the benefit of some mobility, I could get to my home office (which was attached to the garage) and back again—I could become a little more occupied—a little more productive, more useful. Sometime during the third year, Sarah eventually became confident enough to leave me at home alone and go to work for the day, comfort in the knowledge that I could get to a phone and call for help, should the need arise.

After some much needed specialist intervention with my impaired vision, I started learning to drive again. On my second attempt, I passed the mandatory driving test and then things were really looking up. I was just as Shawn was that day back in the hospital therapy clinic; I was driving myself to medical appointments, attending them on my own and reporting back to Sarah when she got home from work. At the same time, I started to spend more time in my office, more time reflecting, more time writing.

Although I did not know it at the time, my journey of reinventing myself had begun in earnest.

FREEDOM (QUEST FOR INDEPENDENCE)

Do you remember climbing that tree on your own?
Or the first time riding your bike—away from home?

Your mum's resignation, "just be home for tea!"
You know … that sensation … when you first became free?

A feeling provided, yet we seldom invoke,
Unless reminded when surviving a stroke.

No more wheelchair, stored away forever,
No more being told, "we must do it together,"

To get in your car and drive to the store,
Making your own decisions, for ever more.

Reliance on others, an unwanted sentence,
Defiance discovered, undaunted independence.

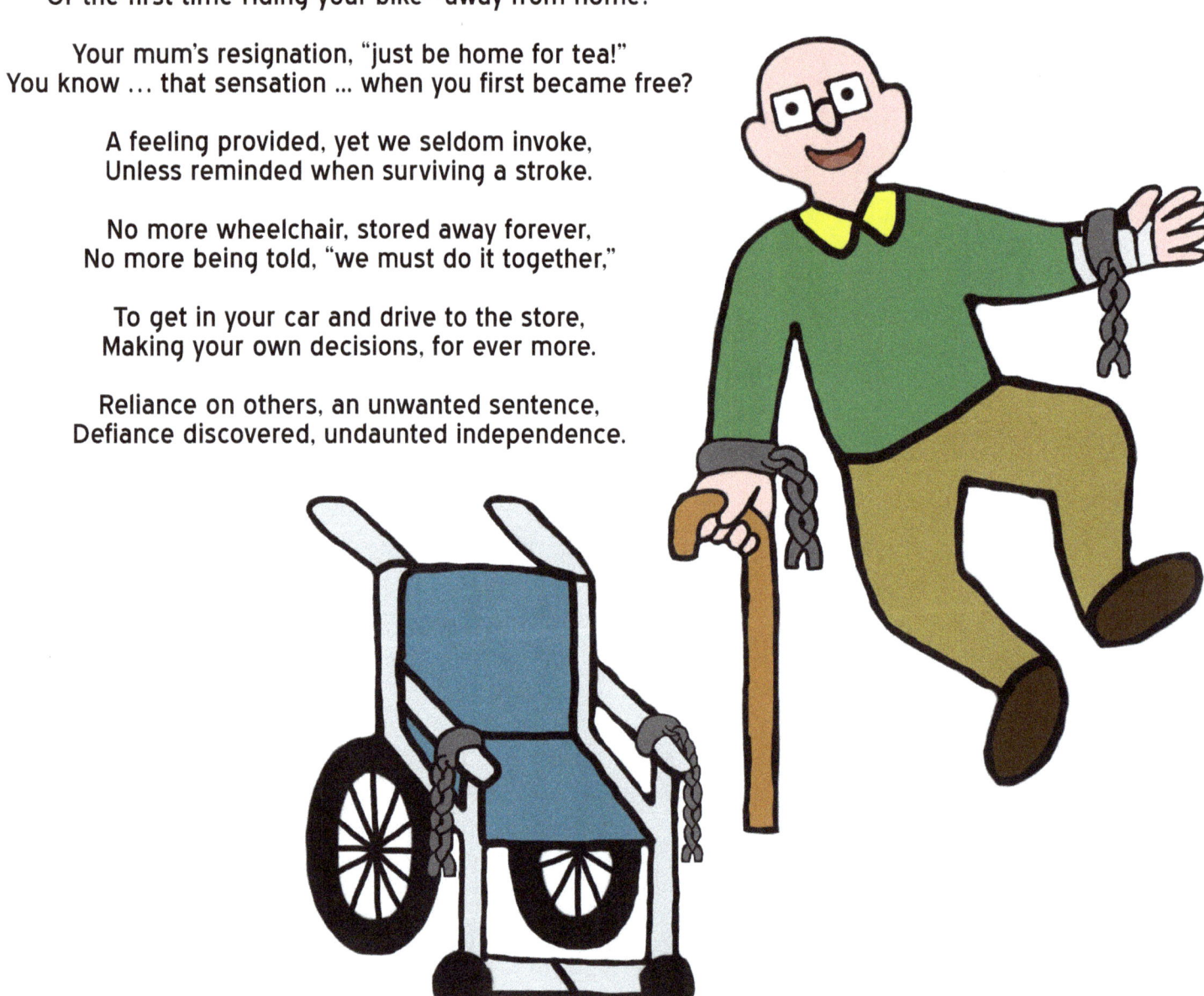

46. PIANO MAN

Following the collapse of my business shortly after the stroke event and the subsequent loss of income, we had to recoup and needed to downsize. Thanks to a lot of help from my visiting sister and brother-in-law, Deborah and Jim, along with a huge amount of paint, we managed to sell our house which served us so well for twenty-five years. We found a very nice smaller single-story home in the town of Wake Forest, around twenty miles northeast of Raleigh and still within commutable distance of RTP.

The area, known as the "Research Triangle Park", was coined because each point is represented by a recognized research university—NC State, Duke, and the University of North Carolina (UNC) of Chapel Hill.

As the more traditional industries of textiles, furniture and agriculture died out, the Research Triangle attracted other employers in the areas of biotechnology and pharmaceuticals as well as microelectronics and information technology. Over the past forty years, the population in the whole area (including Wake Forest) has grown dramatically to the extent that we barely recognize the region since we first moved to North Carolina back in 1994.

It did not take long for me to establish a consistent daily routine which would have me up nice and early each morning; thirty minutes of strenuous stretching exercises followed by a brisk twenty-minute walk (around the block) and after breakfast, I could take Sarah a nice cup of tea before locking myself away in the office.

It was during one of these walks that I met Ronald. It did not take long before we found ourselves walking together, although he was taller and physically stronger than I and one of his strides was the equivalent to about five of mine (it was everything I could do to keep up), he would generously pause at street corners for me to catch my breath and chat a little ...

I sensed that Ronald took pity on me as someone so obviously not from the area and very green about North Carolina life, culture, and overall American history. Ronald had lived in Wake Forest since the day he was born back in 1942 and was very proud of his heritage and quite quick to point out the missing landmarks that had since been demolished to make way for a new street or a new parade of homes. Ronald did not mince his words either and had quite a dim view of people that should know better; "You have never heard of George Washington Carver? You damn fool; when you get home, google him and see!" I was not offended by his pointed recognition of my ignorance; indeed, I was genuinely interested and wanted to learn. Better still, he allowed me to tease him with other informational tidbits that I was a little more familiar and confident (in equal measure and with comparable bluntness). "No way did King James I have sexual relations with his mother! You bloody fool, she left him when he was a baby and she died before he became King of England and Scotland!".

Over coming months, our get-togethers were sporadic and limited to when we bumped into each other but for the most part, quite pleasant and casual. It was only when he told me that he had difficulty getting to places because his car had been out of action for a while, prompting me to offer him a ride, did our association become closer. "That's a mighty loud tail signal you got there, quit using it all the time!" he said one time, prompting me to respond, "I'm doing the driving, it is the way I drive, so tough!" Graciously he would laugh before grunting under his breath, "damn fool!"

I invited him over for tea one afternoon and he told me that his primary doctor did not want to see him unless he was accompanied—she was concerned about his ability to safely drive to the appointment on time and/or to fully appreciate, accept and act on the content of her directions. Ronald asked me if I would like to apply to be his caregiver! Although Ronald is over twenty years my senior, he is definitely more physically mobile and cognitively sharper than me; how he thinks I could possibly help with understanding and even remembering the advice the doctor wanted him to take? I have no idea, but I said I promised to do my best. In quite a short space of time, and many subsequent afternoon cups of tea, and visits with doctors etc., our friendship continued to blossom.

I learned that despite a life full of events his overall ethical code along with his political and spiritual leanings were in tune with mine and I found myself looking forward to his visits and conversational exchanges with relish.

Like many of us, Ronald thinks he is a flawed man and wholeheartedly believes that he has been "spared by the Lord Almighty", as he puts it, and is determined to pay it all back with interest. In this respect, he embarked on a mission to teach young children the piano, music theory, and overall appreciation of music in general, free of any charge. "Sadly, today's education system does not appreciate the value of teaching young children music", he says, "music is the mind expressed in tone" and goes on, "a child who is taught music theory along with mastering a musical instrument will not only benefit from an appreciation of ALL music genres but will perform educationally at a higher level than their peers who do not have the same opportunity," and concluding, "the bible invites worshippers to sing with the Lord, to play an instrument of some kind, clap hands, bang a drum or even crash cymbals together", in short, "to outwardly express our inner-most feelings!"

Naturally, I was very quick to sign up my granddaughter, Lily, to experience and benefit from his tutelage and mentorship. I know in years to come; it will be an experience she will remember with great fondness and gratitude.

I had the good fortune to be near to Ronald the same day the "Arts Wake Forest" organization called him up and invited him to perform at their annual event called "Neck of The Woods" the following month—a small concert series designed to promote local talent. I was delighted to encourage him to accept the honor and even more thrilled to help him short-list the material he would perform which ended up being as diverse as singing a couple of gospel numbers intertwined with two instrumental pieces as challenging as Scott Joplin and Frédéric Chopin could create. The physical and mental effort required to play Chopin's "Polonaise in A Major", is hard enough for someone half his age! Add in a sore shoulder and a tingling left hand (remnants of a car accident eighteen months earlier) and he needed a cheerleader to push him along—a hat I was very happy and honored to wear! The icing on the cake was for Sarah and I to get "front row seats" and witness his exemplary performance that day.

Ronald F. Williams has led an extraordinary life—a life full of twists and turns, downs and ups.

He was forced to take piano lessons at four, married at eighteen, imprisoned at thirty and won a BA in Music from an accredited university at the age of 50—the same age he had his fifth child and along with the other four, a very proud father of them all!

A life that a professionally written, biographical book could not possibly do justice, and at the very least, a book that would likely end up on the fiction shelf!

I only hope that by devoting this one small chapter to him will raise an eyebrow or two of deserved recognition.

PIANO MAN

A mothers' sixth sense, where only she can know,
Making him take lessons on the piano,
Reluctant at first; thought he knew it all,
Failing to appreciate, it was his maker's call,
And so he rose, when others would fall,

Through those early years, he caressed those keys,
A born-again-Mozart, born to please,
Exemplifying expertise.
And thanking the Lord on bended knees,

He conquered Beethoven, Debussy, and Chopin,
At just Eighteen, he became a Piano Man,
Classical, rock, soul; it's no matter,
Hymns all jazzed up for the Lord, to flatter,

Headhunted by a local band,
To become everyone's Piano Man,

He's a teacher, performer; he's that man with a plan,
He's my friend, my mentor; and my, Piano Man.

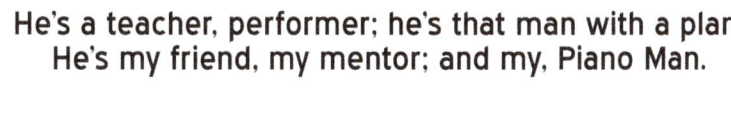

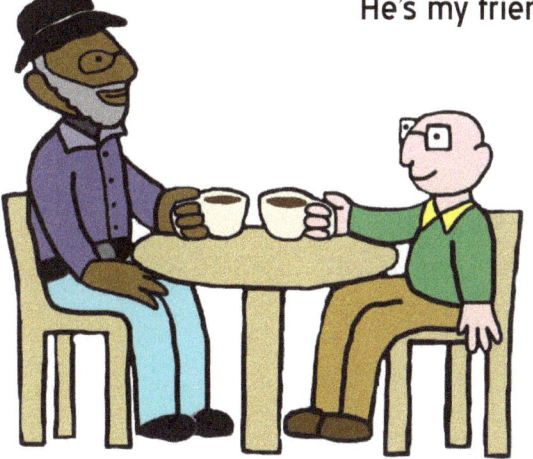

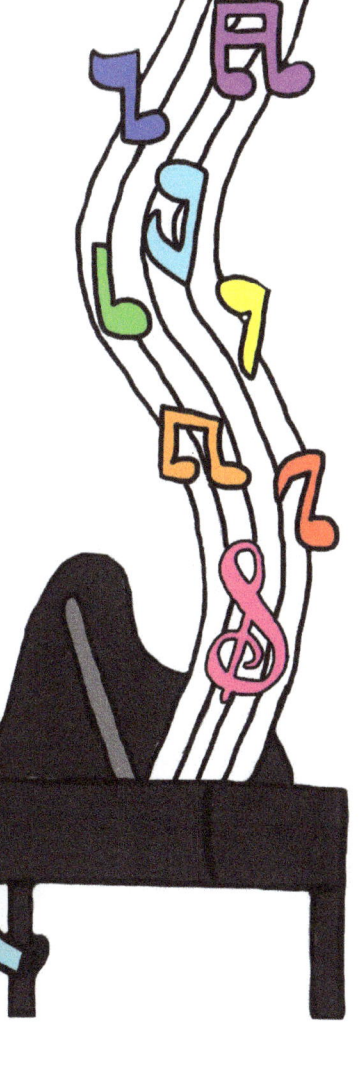

47. LOTTERY

I have a confession to make ... I play the state's lottery game, "Powerball", most weeks!

My failure to have adequately planned our retirement was exacerbated by the fact that I had not envisioned retiring so soon and I had zero contingency for any kind of medical catastrophe, like a stroke. Add in the fact that the aftermath of the stroke left me unable to seek any kind of alternative employment and the amount I earn with the few hours I might do with some subcontract engineering consultancy along with my writing exploits is so inconsequential; you must forgive me for looking elsewhere for some other means of financial reward.

Besides, life is a lottery—some of us get lucky and others not so lucky. I was lucky to have survived my stroke so maybe I can be lucky again?

My former business was doing pretty well at the time of its demise and Sarah and I had hoped to be in a position to sell up one day and afford the ability to purchase a small home back in England, especially as our children had moved on and are making lives for themselves.

Before leaving for America, we sold our house and moved everything over, other than a small pension from my younger years, we have nothing of great tangible worth there anymore, but there are many things we miss let alone the fact that both of us have a number of close relatives and friends of our generation (and older) all very much alive and kicking! And any opportunity to meet with them at their local pub is something worth playing the lottery for, I felt.

Since our move here around twenty-five years ago, property prices in England have inflated by as much as three hundred percent and we have not seen a comparable increase in North Carolina. It will take the size of a lottery win to realize our dream retirement even if we limited our search to a tiny, one bedroom abode in the middle of nowhere, hence my desire to dream and play the lottery!

The main reason for my "confession", is that despite the half of my brain that (sort of) works, I do still consider myself as a rationally minded sort of guy and I am quite capable of understanding what "1:292 million odds" means and that I have a better chance of being struck down by lightning than winning the lottery, but with that said, I still believe in Santa Claus and I also believe in miracles, extraordinary things can happen and I figure the pleasure I get from dreaming about a nice outcome sometime in the future is worth the couple of bucks it costs to play each week.

Of all the arguments against playing the lottery, the best was delivered by my friend Ronald recently. We were driving together on the way to church one Sunday, when I said, "excuse me Ronald but I need to make a brief detour via the gas station and get myself a lottery ticket", after asking me, "what do you want to do that for?" I replied with my usual lame reasoning, only for him to respond with "you damn fool, you already won the lottery—THREE TIMES OVER!".. He went on, "you're alive right?" You got a great family, right? And, you got me as a friend, right? So why would you be so stupid to give your money to the lottery when you already got more than many? AND you can give the money to the church instead!" Naturally, I could not beat that argument, so I chose to shut up and put the money in the collection tray an hour later. I never had the courage to tell Ronald that I picked up a ticket the next day driving home from therapy.

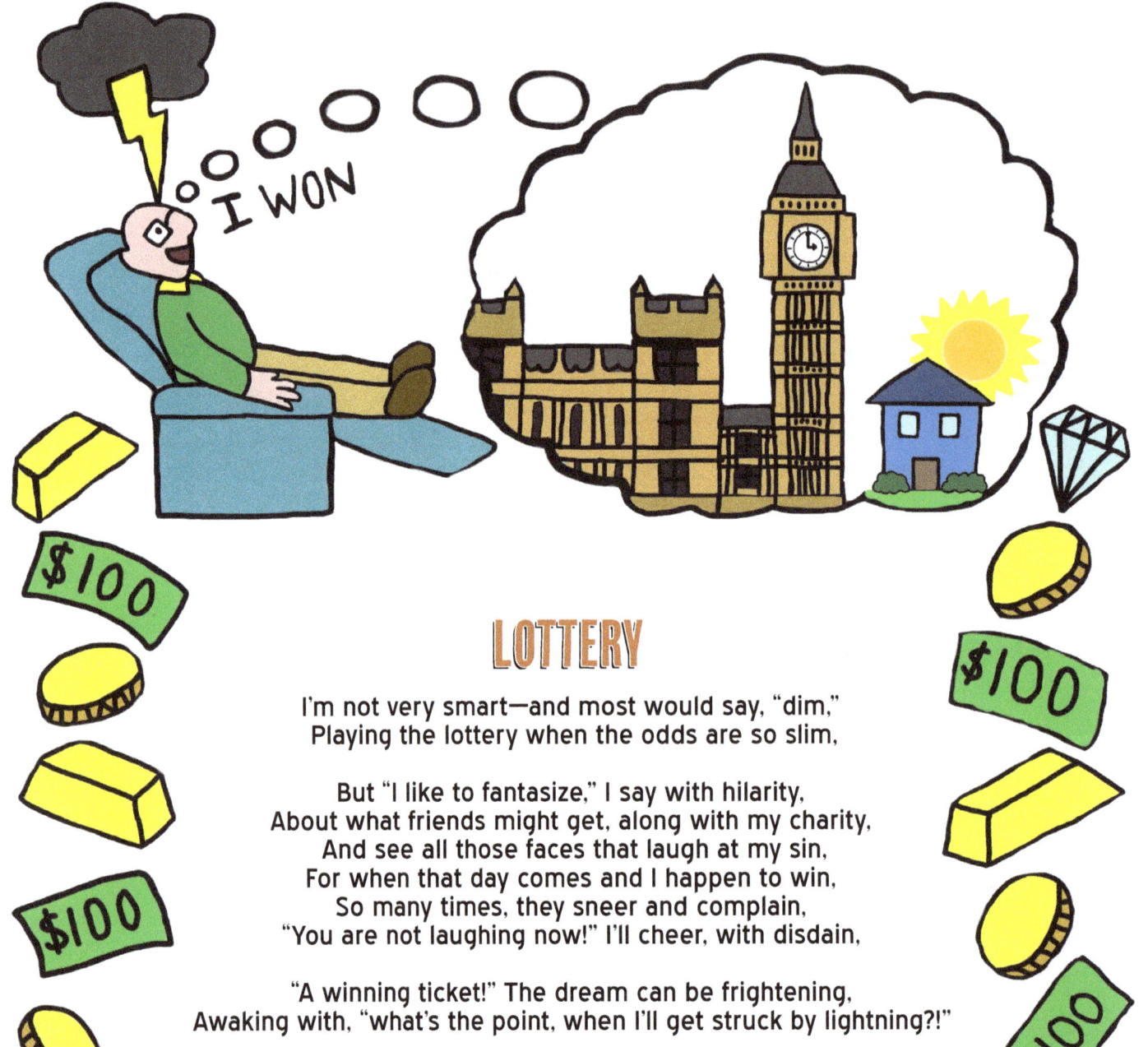

LOTTERY

I'm not very smart—and most would say, "dim,"
Playing the lottery when the odds are so slim,

But "I like to fantasize," I say with hilarity,
About what friends might get, along with my charity,
And see all those faces that laugh at my sin,
For when that day comes and I happen to win,
So many times, they sneer and complain,
"You are not laughing now!" I'll cheer, with disdain,

"A winning ticket!" The dream can be frightening,
Awaking with, "what's the point, when I'll get struck by lightning?!"

48. ACCEPTANCE

This chapter along with the following poem had been a consideration of mine for some time before this book was even on the horizon, and frankly, having read some of my past reflections, ramblings and rantings; this central theme applies pretty much all the way through.

Accepting my circumstance, situation, and limitations, I believe, has made me a better and much happier person; and in my case, a better and happier person than I was even before the stroke! The same can be said to other areas of life in general, so instead of this background being a pleasant introduction to the poem, I feel the need to let off a little steam!

In one of the TAP groups I belong to, we were assigned a book to read called Identity Theft—Rediscovering Ourselves After Stroke by Debra Meyerson PhD … Ms. Meyerson is a Professor of Education at Stanford University and she had suffered a severe (Left hemisphere) stroke which not only caused hemiplegia (to her right-side limbs) but she had the added problem of aphasia as well—which for someone who lectures for a living, was particularly devastating. The story about her recovery journey was both informative and entertaining and I would recommend it to anyone closely connected with the stroke recovery process (survivors, family and friends and other professionals).

She, like me, like many others, worked very hard on therapy treatments with the single-minded determination to recover to where she was before the stroke; she really wanted to get back to work and at the same time, to enjoy participating in family events and outdoor activities, as she did previously. Following many setbacks and frustrations from missed goals she concluded that it was better for her to let go and (reluctantly) accept her disabilities and instead of asking "Who am I now?" Her focus changed to, "Who do I want to become now?" She has since become an advocate and an authority on stroke recovery and particularly, an "aphasia awareness activist", as she puts it; accordingly, she managed to create a new identity for herself that has been satisfying and very rewarding. On more than one occasion Debra states "I am a happier person now". If this sentiment is good enough for a recognized intellect and scholar, then it is certainly good enough for me!

As I have repeatedly suggested, life is not fair, your team does not always win, we don't always get the president we hoped for, and some of us suffer a life changing event, like a stroke.

Get over it, "brush yourself off" and move on with what you have—you will be so much better off for accepting the situation than dealing with the destructive and negative thoughts associated with failing to meet goals along with regret and spite. Although the following poem is tailored more toward the stroke survivor, I do believe the core sentiment applies to everyone/anyone that has experienced a major disappointment of some kind.

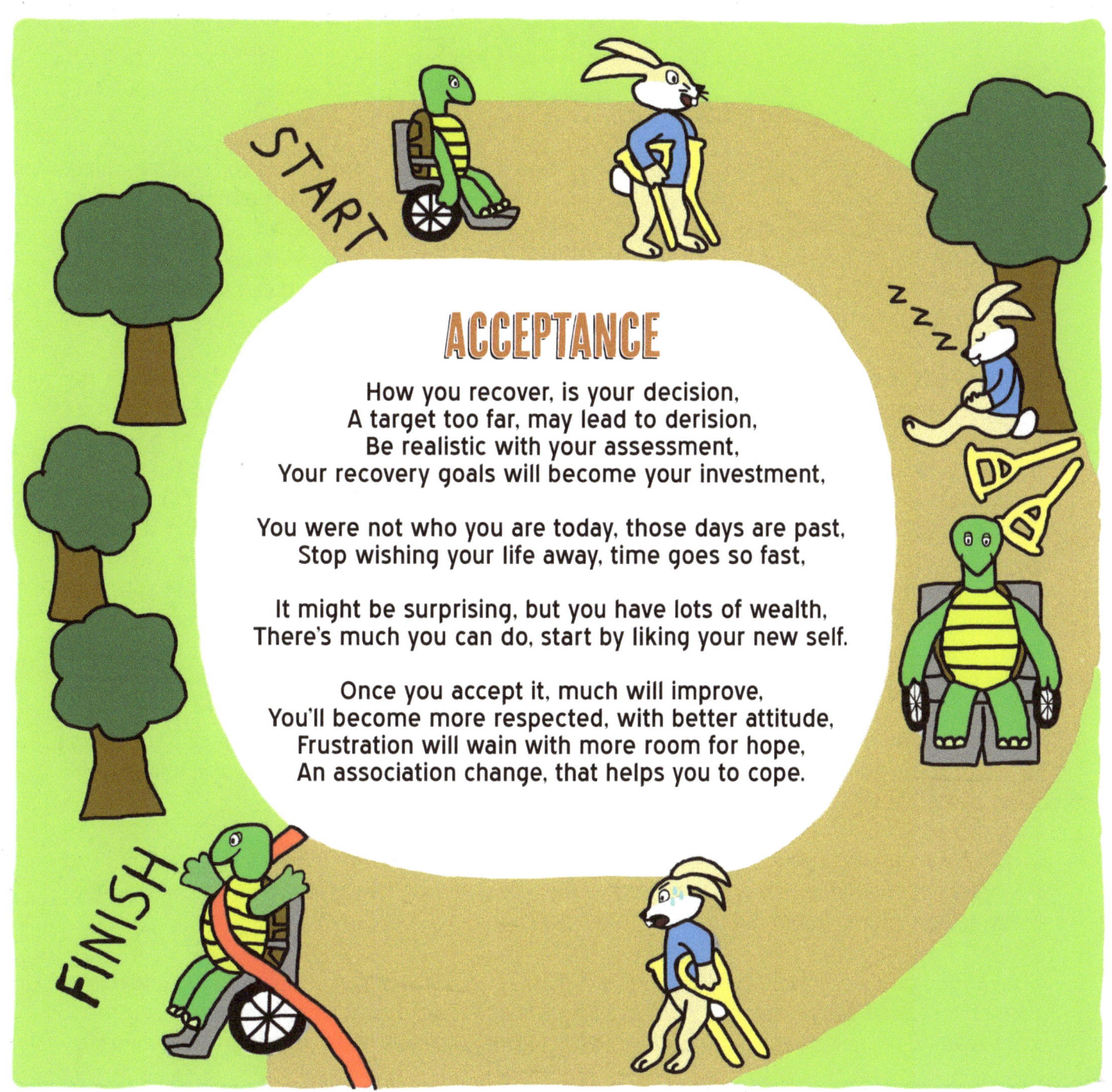

49. REINVENTION

Initially, and considering how I used to push myself, I was quite determined to beat this thing; to get back to how I was before the stroke. But it seemed the more I tried, the more I failed and the more frustrated, angry and short-tempered I would become. It took a while, but after failing at so many things, I eventually concluded that we don't actually "recover" at all, at least not to pre stroke levels; this "recovery journey" we have been told we are taking can be a misleading phrase and for me, is better to describe it as a "journey of discovery".

Through trial and error, I came to learn that it was better for me to unconditionally accept my condition, complete with my new-found disabilities, "warts and all," and search for a new role that could satisfy my needs. Simply put, to move on with what I have got and let go of the things I no longer have. Holding a golf club and playing the guitar would be best placed on the backburner for a while. We may have to hire someone to help with some of the DIY chores I used to do comfortably. My physical pursuits will be limited to the rigorous stretching exercises and a walk around the block each morning and simply resign myself to watching golf and tennis on the TV when one of those big events come around. But, bottom line, my brain still (sort of) functions; I can type with one hand and pursue my writing and undertake some simple engineering consultancy; I can drive a car and get about, participate in activities outside the house without depending upon Sarah. I am quite independent; ultimately, I have a lot going for me; there is much I can do! I concluded that I can be happy over the next few years focusing my attention on my new self. I am very confident that keeping up with my daily exercise routine(s) my left side limbs will progress, but it won't be to the capability before the stroke, and it won't be an overnight thing. C'est La vie! (Which in French means, "tough poo!").

As I got closer with other stroke survivors observing their own journey's regressions and progressions, I came to learn that for many, including myself, it was not about how we were surviving, but more about how we were now thriving.

As an added precaution, and to help prepare for this reflection, I took it upon myself to undertake a small survey of stroke survivor friends and have them complete a simple, self-assessment score relating to their progress on a variety of the issues we now face. The score recorded was in the form of a percentage at various periods of their post stroke journey. The poll revealed that even after 5 years, that most of us never achieved 100% recovery in any of the symptom-categories offered but our optimism regarding our overall future health and wellbeing was on a par or sometimes exceeded our pre-stroke perceptions. In summary, we were content with where we were at, we had survived and got over the trauma associated with stroke. We had learned to move on.

Reinventing myself has helped me to appreciate that it is much better to be flawed and felicitous than overly motivated and morose, as I was in danger of becoming.

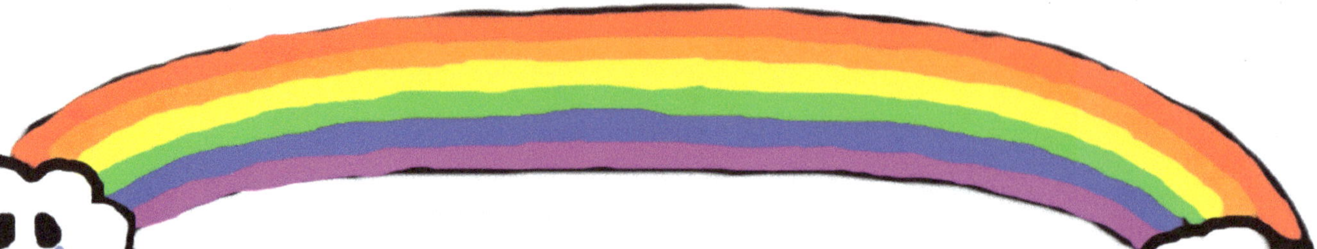

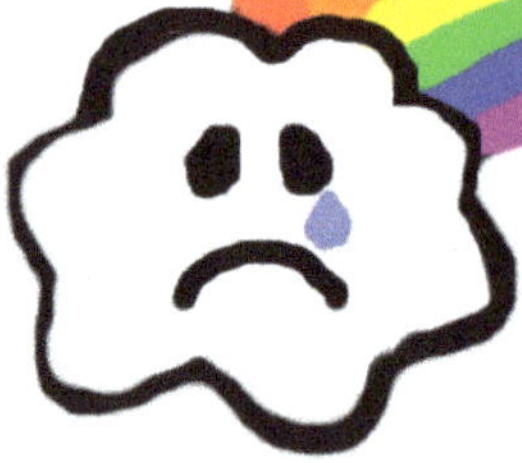

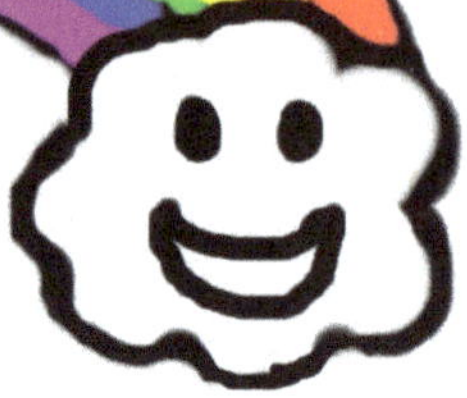

REINVENTION

I did not pick to be the man I am now,
He sneaked up when I was distracted,
It's not been quick, but I have come to learn how,
It is better just to accept him,

Accept him, I have, but giving full attention,
To embrace his strengths the best I can and call it reinvention.

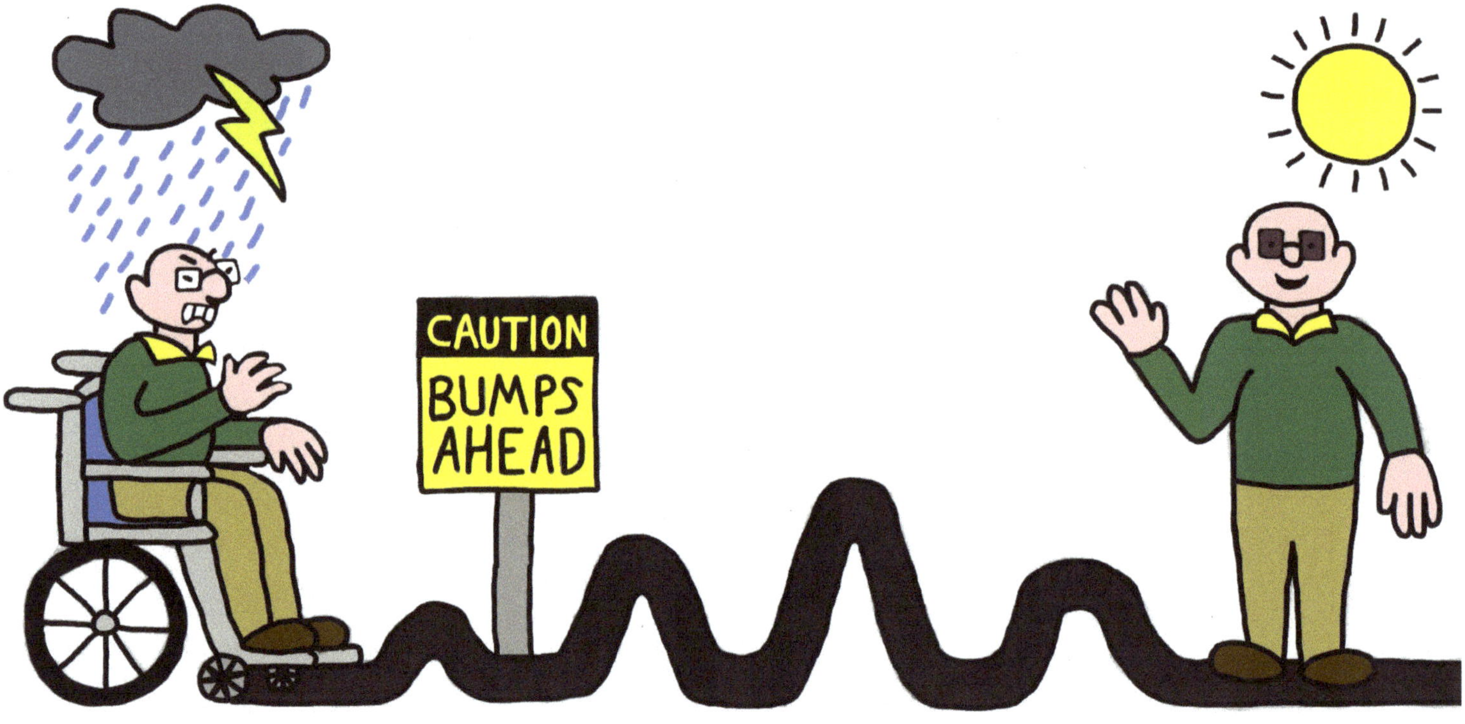

50. BLESSING

One of the best perks of raising a family, is the Sunday family dinner; sitting around the table and catching up on each member's events since we last all sat down together. Our three have all grown up, moved on and made lives for themselves, which makes the fewer times that we do get the chance to gather around the table nowadays, that much more special.

The enjoyment of the family gathering is even greater now considering the experience I have had with surviving the stroke initially and the journey of discovery since. It allows me to appreciate how truly lucky I am.

Without exception, our kids are quite gregarious and have no issues with wearing their hearts on their sleeves and the resulting conversations are quite full of interest—sometimes a little bit of concern when it has been a tough time but invariably entertaining as they recount a situation that was particularly newsworthy.

Now that we have three grandchildren to squeeze around the table it seems we are all competing for the loudest laugh. I cannot say that when I was a young boy and told we were going over to Nanna and Grandpa's house for Sunday roast that I was particularly excited by the prospect; me and my siblings were read the riot act well before we even left the house; our hands were checked for cleanliness, our shoes had to be glistening, even my tie was scrutinized for the knot shape and that the length met with my belt buckle perfectly. We were told exactly how we were going to behave, to keep our voices down and to smile a lot; basically, how we were going to be angelic and definitely, not to let our parents down. We were going to say "please" and "thank you" at every opportunity; we will remain clean and tidy throughout the visit and how we will portray children that appreciated every morsel that was placed on our plates; oh, and be sure to ask at the appropriate times … "can I help wash the dishes Nanna?" and, "can you play something on the organ Grandpa?" Grandpa was a very good musician, but it wasn't the sort of music I particularly wanted to hear at my age … I would have much rather asked, "can you put on the TV please? (There is a really good western/movie starring John Wayne)."

Now that my role has reversed and I have earned my place at the head of the table, I appreciate the sense of pride my parents and grandparents must have felt and equally, the disappointment when the occasion does not rise to expectations.

The following blessing is designed to help prepare and remind the party what it is all about — I should point out that it is not guaranteed to work every time!

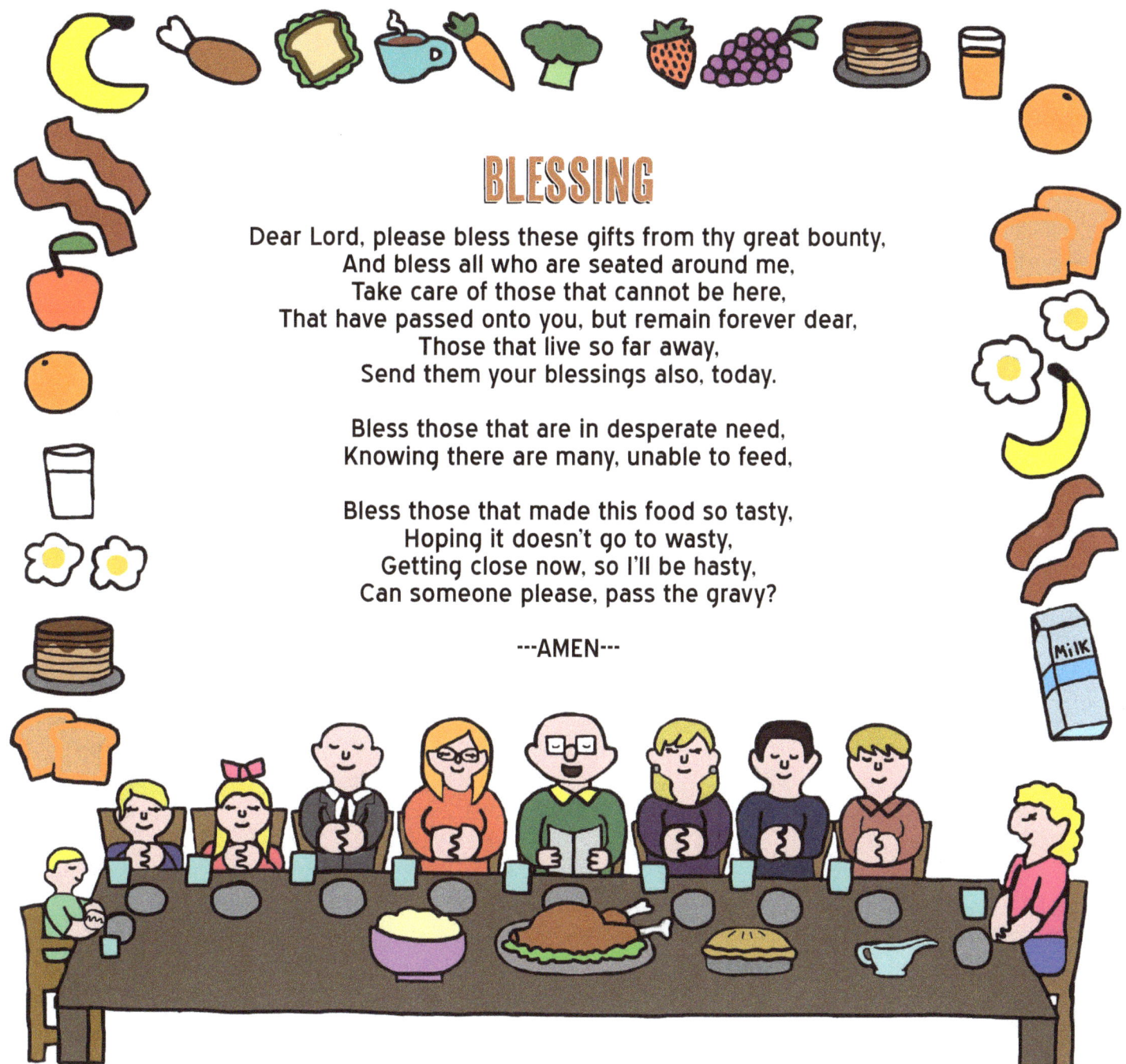

51. BULLDOG

In 2002, the BBC conducted a poll of the British public to determine "the top one hundred Britons in history".

Leading the list, was the former Prime Minister and Statesman, Sir Winston Churchill (1874-1965); other notables included, Isaac Newton, Alexander Fleming, and Charles Darwin as top scientists along with William Shakespeare, Charles Dickens, and John Lennon from the arts, music and literary community. Winston had some tough competition.

Since 2002 and subsequent opinion polls, Winston Churchill is consistently found in the top three of these popularity contests as the most highly revered Briton to ever walk our "green and pleasant land" (as referenced by William Blake, the poet that created the phrase in his poem, "Jerusalem" —a poet that only got to thirty-eighth on the list back in 2002, I might add).

Of course, these polls can be very subjective and depending on the maturity of the voter, open to considerable conjecture! After all, the original poll, had in its top fifty, the likes of David Beckham, Tony Blair, Guy Fawkes and Boy George, which rather lowers the tone, somewhat! But then, I am an old "conservative, fuddy-duddy".

Sidney Strube (1891-1956) was an established cartoonist working for the Daily Express newspaper at the time and was the first (in June. 1940) to depict Churchill as some kind of therianthropic bulldog in a combative posture almost daring the Nazi's to fight him, and this image stuck to the extent that the analogy would recur in hundreds more caricatures during those (Second world War) years.

It so happens that I have always been a massive fan of Winston Leonard Spencer Churchill, his accomplishments, his role in the defeat of Nazi-fascism in the Second World War and particularly, his sharp wit and raconteurial character in general.

Poststroke, I have tended to relate to him even more since I see a number of parallels between us —understanding of course, the proportions are significantly skewed in his favor.

Addressing the major differences first; Churchill was born into the British aristocracy as the eldest son of Lord Randolph Churchill and Jenny Jerome, and the paternal grandson of the seventh Duke of Marlborough. I have absolutely no "blue blood" running through my veins! Further, Winston was privately educated before moving to a military school at Sandhurst. My parents recognized quite early on not to waste their hard-earned money on my education and my only knowledge of the military is that you hold a rifle opposite and away from the pointy end!

Churchill was both a citizen of the United Kingdom and the United States although unlike me, the latter for him was bestowed as a (one and only) honorary citizenship from a grateful President John F. Kennedy in 1963. Further, Winston's mother, Jenny Jerome, was born in New York thus making him half American (by blood) anyway.

Nobody could deliver a riposte better than Winston Churchill; reportedly, Lady Nancy Astor once said to him:" Winston, if I were your wife, I would poison your tea!" prompting his response, "Nancy, if I were your husband, I would drink it!" I wish I had the audacity and sharpness of mind and the presence to get away with such a retort, but frankly, Winston Churchill was way out of my league.

On the other hand, like me, Winston Churchill was not a model student, he got bored quite easily with work that did not interest him (which has always been my excuse), but we both managed to scrape by enough to graduate into a career of some kind.

Churchill famously said, "To make water palatable, we had to add whiskey and by diligent effort, I learned to like it." Unfortunately for us both not only did we enjoy a tipple or two but we both smoked as well. Both vices are on top of the "How NOT to avoid a stroke" list, accordingly, we both suffered strokes—although typically, he beat me in quantity, (at least by) six to one.

Despite having his first major stroke in 1949, Churchill rebounded back onto the political scene winning the general election and reinstatement of his premiership in 1951; sadly, another stroke in 1953 would cause him to resign in favor of his deputy, Anthony Eden.

Drawing on his early years as a military journalist, Churchill continued his writing to the extent that between the ages of 79 and 90 (at the time of his death in 1965) he wrote and published a further five literary works, one of which, Defending Exalted Human Values won him a Nobel Prize for literature. Again, very few can compare with him and least of all, me!

I had originally proposed this chapter and poem be titled "Short Fat Bald Guy", playing on that similarity between us, only to find as I researched Churchill further, he was 2 inches taller than I. It is easy to think of him as shorter man—he was 71 years old when he first became Prime Minister and nearly 80 years old when he left office on his second go around; it is understandable to think of him as being short as the cameras filmed him "stooping" about the place with his walking stick in hand. I was born plump and short and remained so all of my life much to my mother's regret.

Against normal protocol for non-royals, Winston Leonard Spencer Churchill was honored with a state funeral. "Operation Hope Not" was initiated and planned the moment he left public office in 1953 and went into action on January 26, 1965 (2 days after he died) and by decree from Queen Elizabeth, his body lay in state at Westminster for three days (23 hours per day) before the funeral service proper. Over 320,000 members of the public waited up to three hours in a line often one mile long to pay their respects. The funeral service was held at St. Paul's Cathedral on the following Saturday, January 30, 1965, attended by the Queen, many heads of state and high-ranking representatives from 112 countries. It was said to be the largest state funeral in history.

After the service, the coffin was taken to the Tower of London, and following a 19-gun salute, placed on a launch which then sailed up the river Thames where sixteen RAF fighter jets flew overhead, and thirty-six dock cranes "bowed" their jibs as the vessel passed by. Members of Churchill's family joined him for the river ride before catching a special train from Waterloo that would take them to the Oxfordshire village of Bladon and St Martin's Church where he was laid to rest within his (Marlborough) family plot alongside his ancestors. On route, at the stations and in the fields, many thousands of people that could not get down to London also came out to offer their final farewells as the train whistled by.

I don't suppose many of us were in London at the time to witness the spectacle; however, there is a very good, summarized (five minute) movie available on the Worldwide Web you can watch. Simply type "Winston Churchill—I vow to thee" in your search engine box and it should become available for viewing; and if you are a fan like me, I recommend you have a tissue handy before watching!

BULLDOG

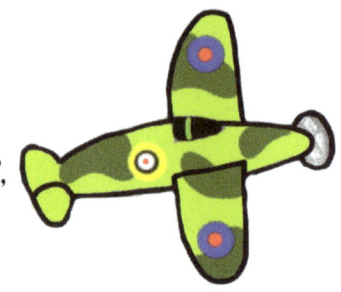

Before Berlin capitulated,
His concerns were clearly stated,
His writings strewn large and "on the wall",
And very soon, France would fall,

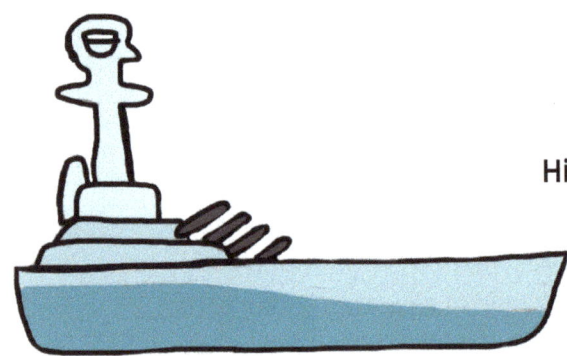

Refusing to negotiate,
'Twas his destiny and the world's fate,
"We are next!" he prophesied,
And with everything, they tried,
Motivating "the few" to the skies,
Who cut them off in their stride,

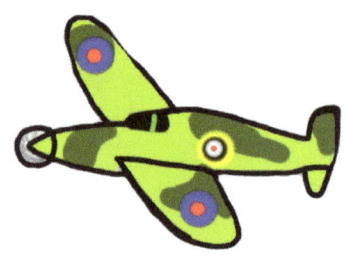

His writing skills and those speeches,
Inviting us to the hills,
and on those beaches,

He said, it was "the end of the beginning,"
But this was just his first inning,
A simple lust to keep on winning,

The stroke would smirch but no great burden,
For he unearthed, as he knew for certain,
The wicked scourge, behind that curtain.

Thousands came to say goodbye,
To espouse and claim the "Bulldog", their pugnacious guy,
No surprise, no wonder why.

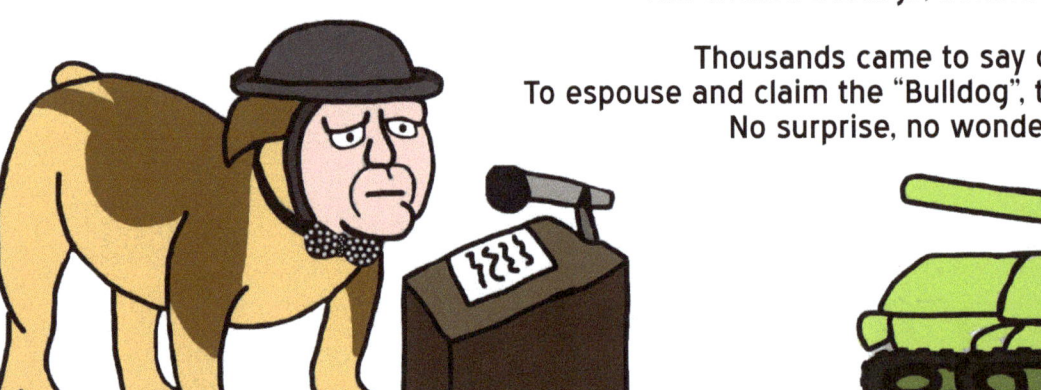

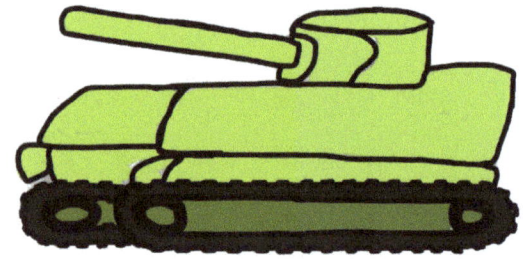

BAD RHYMES, NO REASON

52. ORIGINS

My first book's manuscript was completed in July 2018 and the book was published six months later in January 2019.

I had no job to go to and I needed to keep myself busy before considering another book. I needed to keep my brain active.

After my mother's passing and having gone through the many photos she left behind, it occurred to me that despite the great privilege of knowing both pairs of grandparents and various great uncles and aunts very well along with the few stories they passed down to me, nothing was properly documented and there were still a number of holes in our family history that I did not know and very few (living) sources I could go to, to access the information.

It seems that it is only after the passing of a parent/grandparent, do we regret the many conversational opportunities we could have had with them and that we did not delve a little deeper into their own family memories.

My granddaughter was approaching her sixth birthday and it occurred to me that my gift to her could be a framed family tree poster for her bedroom wall showing her family lineage – on both sides of the pond. And with the help of my daughter in law's parents, living and older members of our respective families and a couple of online facilities, I set about the process of researching her family genealogy. For someone in my condition especially with my level of focus, the exercise was extremely challenging and demanding, but above all, absorbing and highly rewarding! It took me about six months to compile, and the final chart contained well over six hundred family members—most of which, I was not previously familiar, and where, on my mother's side I could go back to the seventeenth century and on Sarah's paternal line, all the way back to the sixteenth! Indeed one of the many highlights was the discovery that Sarah is directly related (through 12 generations) to a Mr. Nathaniel Hancock (1596-1652), who, as a young adult and like so many, set sail from England for the "New World", married a Ms. Joanna Wright (1612-1652) in Cambridge, MA and between them, they would become the great-grandparents of Mr. John Hancock (1737-1793), the first Governor of Massachusetts, a recognized Founding Father and the most conspicuous signature on the Declaration Of Independence.

There is a wealth of information available if you care to look. In the UK, our church/parish records (births, baptisms and deaths) are quite comprehensive and go back through the centuries. Britons have been obliged to complete census surveys for many decades. These censuses would provide the address of the abode, the "head of the household", spouse and each child; and every line entry would include full name of the occupant, their age, place of birth along with their occupation. We can guess the hardships and adventures they had based on the standard of living and surroundings of their time.

I am so grateful that my mother kept and protected the photos she had, since they provide a small glimpse of our long-departed relative(s) and how they appeared. But for those living prior to the mid-nineteenth century, before the popular photographic era, we can only guess. My great (x12) grandfather Cardno (1620-1703) and Sarah's Great (x9) Uncle John Hancock had the means and notoriety to justify portraiture, at least.

This exercise also reminded me how fortunate we are to be living in a period with all the major medical advances we now enjoy. Very rarely did I find family members before my grandparents' generation living beyond the age of 75.

I could not find evidence of any members within our family ancestry had suffered a stroke and I am sure, that pre-1900, the chances were remote that one could survive the ordeal.

In my case, the blood clot that traveled from the heart to my brain occurred during a weekday when I was on the phone in my office, I was extremely lucky to have survived. First, because one of my staff found me quite soon after collapsing to the floor, second that he happened to be a former paramedic and recognized my symptoms and could relay them onto the emergency services; third because the paramedics arrived very quickly; lastly and most importantly, I was rushed to a hospital that had only recently introduced an emergency stroke response program along with the establishment of a specialist stroke care team. Upon my arrival to the emergency room, the resident doctor undertook a preliminary examination and suspecting the cause immediately had me undergo various brain scans and imagery which was made available to the on-call neurologist and due to the fact that barely three hours had passed I was prescribed "tPA" (Tissue Plasminogen Activator) - a quite revolutionary (tried and tested) "clot-busting" drug that would help clear the blockage. I was then treated and kept in ICU under the watchful eye of the neurologist and highly trained nursing staff with regular scans to monitor the progress of my overly swollen brain. In short, many do not survive a stroke either through absence of diagnosis or more likely, reaction time was too little, too late.

Examples of well-known people that were not so fortunate as me go back as far as; Johann Sebastian Bach suspected of passing due to stroke all the way back in 1750 at the age of 65. Ironically, all three leaders of the allied powers during World War 2 met their demise at the hands of a stroke starting with Franklin D. Roosevelt in 1945 at the age of 63, Joseph Stalin in 1953 at the age of 74 and finally, Winston Churchill in 1965 at 90 years old (although this was his third "massive" stroke on record). The 37th US President, Richard Nixon also died from a stroke in 1994 at the age of 81. In fact, there are many notable Politicians (to many to mention) that died from stroke. Famous Celebrities include the actress Grace Kelly, at just 52 years old, that had a stroke when she lost control of her car when driving back to her country estate in Monaco in 1982. Her co-star in "To Catch a Thief", Cary Grant, had his stroke in 1986 at the age of 82. Just one day after the news of her daughter, Carrie Fisher's, sudden death in 1982, the Hollywood Singer and Dancer, Debbie Reynolds died from a hemorrhagic stroke at the age of 84. Her co-star in "Singing in The Rain", Gene Kelly died from a stroke in 1996, he was 83 years old. It would appear that it is not just an age or era thing; Bill Paxton was just 61 when his stroke killed him in 2017 and Luke Perry had the same (ischemic) stroke at the same age I had mine as recently as 2019. Yet, he died whereas I survived. I don't know the rhyme or reason, but I feel I was particularly lucky that day back in May 2013.

Who knows, I may still have a few more years (and a couple more books) left in me yet?

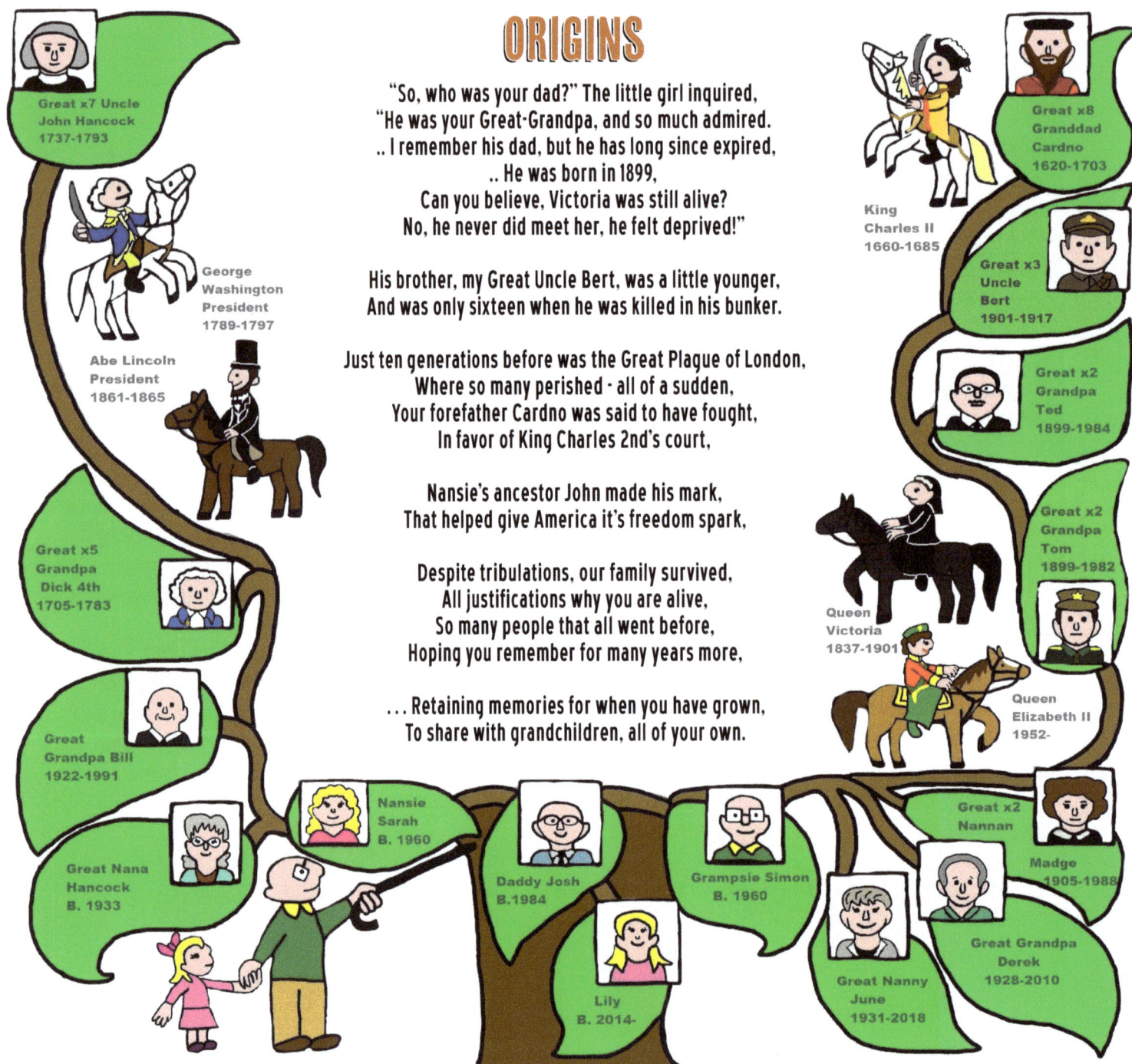

53. GRUMPY OLD FART

As implied on more than one occasion, my poststroke journey (nine and a half years to this date of publication), does not conclude happily with me giving you an impressive, itemized list of the achievements I made, and the recoveries gained. I can tell you that I can walk better than I did last year which was better than the year before. My left arm and hand are less spastic than last year and significantly better than two years ago. For me, the single most important accomplishment has been my overall cognitive wellbeing. Over the past couple of years, I have undertaken some engineering support work quite close to the level(s) I used to achieve—at least my customer(s) have been satisfied enough to pay me for my efforts. Further, I have managed to write two books relating to a subject that just ten years ago, I knew absolutely nothing about and a subject matter that I feel knowledgeable enough to stand in front of an educated audience and speak authoritatively and with confidence.

The single best thing about my journey, as with many inspirational journey type stories (Rocky, Forest Gump, et al.) is that in the case of the stroke survivor, we start our journey as the underdog. Not only was I physically handicapped from the get-go, but I was blind even to where I was going. The journey is nowhere near over yet (and may never be over until I'm six feet under), but through a willingness to accept and reinvent, I am happier and better prepared to take whatever challenges might be thrown my way in the future.

I would even go so far to say that I am better off today than I was before my brain injury almost to the extent, that I think everybody should have a stroke! Although I am not sure Uncle Sam could afford for us all to have one.

Dare I even suggest that Sarah thinks she is having an affair with another man—lucky me!

With all that said, it is only right that I try to assess as best I can, who it is, through the process of reinvention, I have become?

Through the previous chapters and reflections, I feel I have revealed my inner self enough that you have a pretty good idea as to the type of bloke I have morphed into. I am also happy to acknowledge that just because I am happy with me, doesn't mean anyone else has to be—but isn't that what life is about?

As it happens, the experience gained from my first book taught me the importance of "proofreading"—lots of times! Even after my initial due diligence and (supposedly) the publisher-editor's courtesy review, within a couple of months following publication of that first book, I received a number of calls that started along the lines, "On page XY, did you mean to?" So embarrassing. Accordingly, I started proofreading this book long before I got to this last chapter and it became apparent as I read each reflection, that on more than one occasion, the "rantings" got the better of the "ramblings" …

I did forecast, warn, and (sort of) apologize in the preface about the potential, but it was genuinely only through this realization that brought home the type of person I am now (a bit like one of those grandparents we did not like to spend time with). But I am sure, they, like me, were still happy within themselves, and I am okay with that. I contend that regardless of your situation, everyone should ask themselves, "am I happy within myself?

If not, maybe they should try a little reinvention, I recommend it, it worked wonders for me!

I still need to reiterate the one important lesson (that for me, took the longest to learn); that being, no two strokes are the same. If believed, then understandably, no two poststroke journeys will be the same either. I mentioned a stroke survivor that I first met during one of my rehab hospital therapy sessions, Shawn Fleck. Shawn had his stroke event four months before mine, his brain injury was to the left hemisphere, resulting in hemiparesis to his right-side limbs but with the added burden of aphasia which proved to be an enormous (communicative) struggle his first year. But in his case, he has diligently set goals for himself and worked very hard to meet and exceed those goals, starting with his speech and then his mobility issues. We meet for a beer quite regularly and I am often in awe of the extent of the activities he now enjoys (he plays a lot of golf)—although he readily admits he is not fully recovered to pre stroke levels. I would also say that he is as happy in himself as I am with me. But isn't that what makes us human? Some of us get to enjoy and play a good game of golf, others like to devote their time and talents in support of those in need, and some of us would rather stay at home and spend their spare time writing stories.

Ultimately, like so many things, there is no magic pill; there is no right and only way. I only hope that for those that have the misfortune to survive a stroke in the future have access to some good advice. At the earliest opportunity get yourself involved with as many stroke support groups as you can, surround yourself with people fighting similar battles. It is from my own experiences contributed by the many I have come to know and admire that I can summarize and leave you with my top two thoughts:

1. Don't compare yourself with others—your injury, your personal circumstances and your poststroke journey will be quite unique to you.

2. Whilst having a stroke is a leading cause for serious long-term disability, IT IS NOT THE END OF THE WORLD—you survived. Indeed, it is just a beginning of a new chapter in your lives. It will be a very long and mostly uphill journey for you and your loved ones and the sooner you all can come to terms with it and accept that you are unlikely to ever get back everything you lost before the event, the better off you will be. I am sure this mindset has worked for me, and my stroke survivor friends. and the new people we have all been obliged to become.

Regardless, I still felt it might be appropriate to acknowledge the present, my new self, along with my character flaw(s) and conclude the book with that sentiment in a silly rhyme here:

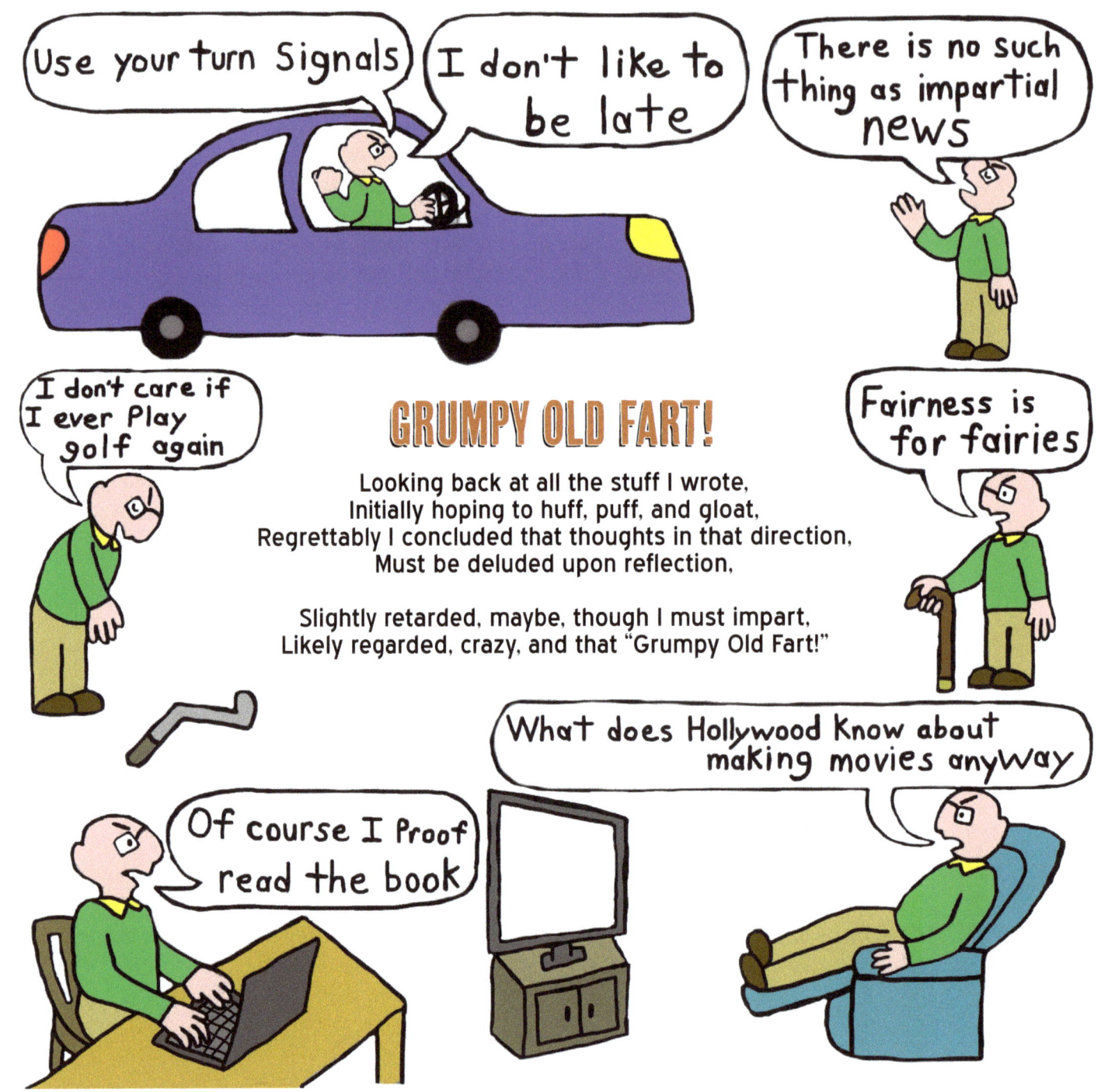

ACKNOWLEDGEMENTS

I must first acknowledge my wife, Sarah, and children, Josh, Luke, and Hannah, for their unswerving support with this venture, accepting my prolonged absences locked away in my office for hours at a time, and particularly for the way they all did a really good job pretending to be impressed with the few sample pages I insisted they read along the way!

A special thanks to my older sister, Deborah Sparham in England. Following my mother's demise and passing; took on the mantle as the family's matriarch, and with pleasure (as she did when we were growing up) rose to the task of kicking me, frequently, to try harder with zero tolerance for self-pity. I am only sorry that I have been unable to give her the "good thrashing" she deserved on the golf course that for a while, we both wanted. With no help from me, she has become Ladies Captain of her local club with a golf handicap that got down to just 16.2 —better than I ever achieved pre stroke. Which makes me wonder, who will be doing the thrashing?

I would like to say a very big thank you to Ms. Maura Silverman MS, CCC/SLP and the Triangle Aphasia Project (TAP) organization she founded along with the many brain injured survivors that make up her "family" of clients, not only for her counsel on technical matters relating to post stroke recovery but the many inspiring journey stories that provided much of the fuel for the content of this work.

I further appreciated the unlimited and free online access I had to the CDC website which provided much of the statistical data referenced.

Last but not least, I must pay special tribute to MPP for believing my manuscript had potential enough to sign me up for a publishing association and then giving me unlimited access to their highly talented editor, Ms. Florence Mayberry, who, with a great deal of patience and oodles of tolerance, somehow found a way to help me take that first (very rough) draft and turn it into something a little more readable and worthy of publication, I could write a book about the learning experience gained!

ABOUT THE AUTHOR

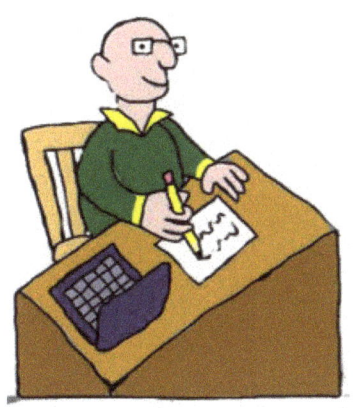

Simon Charles Barton was born and raised about 15 miles southwest of London England, in 1960. He studied and practiced Mechanical Engineering Design before moving to North Carolina with his wife, Sarah and their 3 children in 1994. At the time of his stroke in 2013, he owned and managed his Design and Applications Engineering business in the Triangle Park area of North Carolina, where he still lives today. With the closure of his business in 2015, he took to writing, publishing his first book, *Not so Green as Cabbage Looking*, in 2019.

ABOUT THE ILLUSTRATOR

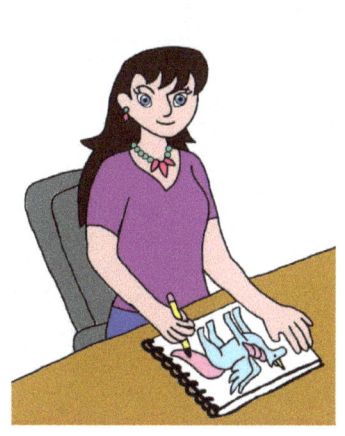

Sarah Constance Hardy was born in Raleigh, NC in 1990. At age four, she was diagnosed as mildly autistic, and her parents were told that she would never function as a normal child. Her parents told her she was very artistic and gave her art lessons and home-schooled her from age twelve onward. At a young age she had a strong interest in dragons, unicorns, and other fantasy creatures from reading books and watching movies. At age fifteen, she started writing stories and created a world where all her favorite magical creatures lived together in harmony. She has now written, illustrated and published two original books — *The Silver Winged Dragon* in 2011 and *The Unicorn and The Pegasus* in 2020.

Simon was "delighted and excited" when Constance accepted his invitation to join him on this project, adding, "I figured that the poems in their own right, were not particularly pleasing to the ear, so my hope was that Constance could make them a little more pleasing to the eye, at least! And in this respect, she has met and exceeded my expectations—I am sure the reader would agree."

www.ingramcontent.com/pod-product-compliance
Lightning Source LLC
Chambersburg PA
CBHW040000290426
43673CB00077B/290